Neuroimaging

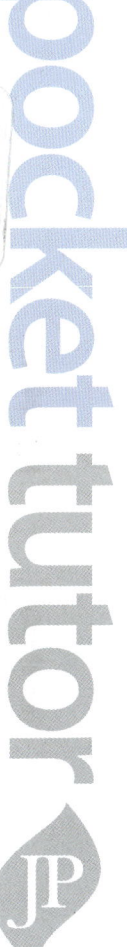

pocket tutor

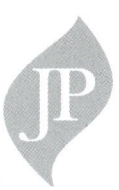

Neuroimaging

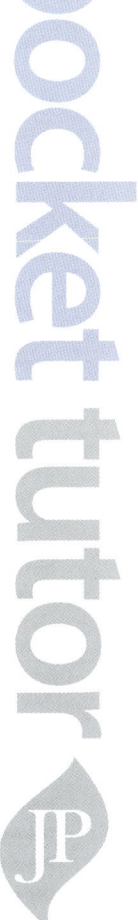

Rory Piper MBChB BMedSci(Hons) MRCS(Ed)
NIHR Academic Clinical Fellow
University of Oxford
Specialty Trainee in Neurosurgery
John Radcliffe Hospital
Oxford, UK

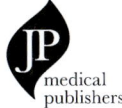
medical
publishers

© 2018 JP Medical Ltd.

Published by JP Medical Ltd, 83 Victoria Street, London, SW1H 0HW, UK

Tel: +44 (0)20 3170 8910   Fax: +44 (0)20 3008 6180

Email: info@jpmedpub.com   Web: www.jpmedpub.com

ISBN: 978-1-909836-57-0

British Library Cataloguing in Publication Data
A catalogue record for this book is available from the British Library

Library of Congress Cataloging in Publication Data
A catalog record for this book is available from the Library of Congress

Publisher:	Richard Furn
Development Editor:	Thomas Banister-Fletcher
Editorial Assistant:	Adam Rajah
Design:	Designers Collective Ltd

Foreword

Brain imaging is a core hospital service: a quarter of all admissions are 'neurological' and most of these patients will have their brains imaged. Every minute lost prior to treatment is thought to represent one million extra brain cells dying, therefore many diagnoses need to be made swiftly in order for the patient to receive the best treatment as soon as possible. This makes the ability to interpret neuroradiological imaging crucial and *Pocket Tutor Neuroimaging* is an excellent portable and accessible guide to the essential knowledge of neuroradiology.

The book opens by describing the main neurological imaging techniques, particularly MRI and CT. The indications, interpretation and protocols for each technique are detailed, with common conditions presented alongside their differential diagnosis and a large number of high-quality images.

The teaching of neuroradiology is frequently haphazard and often missed by students completely. However, it is crucial to have an understanding of neuroradiology; what other specialty will allow you to see what an unconscious patient's brain looks like? So be smart, buy this book and have a real edge on your peers. Even better, use this book to make a real difference to your patients with your speedy and accurate diagnoses.

Robin Sellar
Professor of Neuroradiology
The University of Edinburgh
Edinburgh, UK

Preface

Neuroimaging is encountered across all medical specialties, not only neurology and neurosurgery – from trauma calls in the emergency department to falls in the medicine of the elderly ward, and of course in medical school or postgraduate exams.

Pocket Tutor Neuroimaging is intended for medical students in their clinical years and doctors in the early years of their training. Its aim is to demystify neuroimaging and provide a broad understanding of how to interpret normal and abnormal appearances.

The book opens with a summary of the essential anatomy and describes the different imaging techniques. Next is an introduction to the principles of interpretation of images of the normal and abnormal nervous system. The remaining chapters demonstrate the uses of neuroimaging in disease and they focus on the serious but common pathologies that a junior doctor may encounter. Each one includes at least one case scenario to relate the content back to clinical practice.

I wish you the best of luck in your studies and clinical careers, and I hope that this book will help you along the way.

Rory J Piper
March 2018

Contents

Chapter 9 Spinal conditions

Dedications and acknowledgements

I would like to thank Richard Furn, Thomas Banister-Fletcher and Adam Rajah at JP Medical for all of their hard work and for making this book possible.

Thank you to my wife, Allisyn, for her endless patience and support.

Thank you to the reviewers of the book:
Chapter 1 - Dr Samantha Mills
Chapter 2 - Dr Conal Corbally
Chapter 3 - Dr Paul Burns and Dr Phillip Rich
Chapter 4 - Mr Aimun Jamjoom and Dr Shahriar Islam
Chapter 5 - Dr Grant Mair
Chapter 6 - Dr Mark Rodrigues
Chapter 7 - Dr Gerard Thompson
Chapter 8 - Mr Stephen Price and Dr Harpreet Hayre
Chapter 9 - Mr Rodney Laing and Dr Peter Keston

Lastly, thank you to Professor Sellar for the kind foreword and for the support in the writing process.

RP

Figures 2.10, 2.11, 2.12, 2.14, 2.24, 3.11, 4.9, 5.1, 5.2, 9.2, 9.3 and 9.4 are reproduced from Heir M, Vaidhyanath R. Pocket Tutor Emergency Imaging. London: JP Medical, 2013.

Figures 1.3, 1.59, 1.7, 3.3, 5.10, 5.12, 5.14, 5.15 and 6.3 are reproduced from Collins DR, Goodfellow JA, Silva AHD, et al. Eureka Neurology & Neurosurgery. London: JP Medical, 2016.

First principles

An understanding of neuroimaging rests on knowledge of the fundamental principles of:
- neuroanatomy (the structure of the normal brain)
- neuroimaging terminology (how images are described)
- neuroimaging modalities (how images are acquired)
- safety in neuroimaging

1.1 Neuroanatomy

The nervous system is divided into:
- A central nervous system and
- A peripheral nervous system

This book focuses on the central nervous system, which comprises the brain and spinal cord.

The scalp

The scalp is the soft tissue covering the skull vault. A mnemonic for the five layers that make up the scalp, from superficial to deep, is SCALP:
- **S**kin
- **C**onnective tissue
- **A**poneurosis (the galea aponeurotica)
- **L**oose areolar connective tissue
- **P**eriosteum (pericranium)

The skull

The skull is divided into:
- The neurocranium, i.e. the part encasing the brain, and
- The viscerocranium, i.e. the facial skeleton

The neurocranium

The neurocranium forms the cranial cavity, the space occupied by the brain.

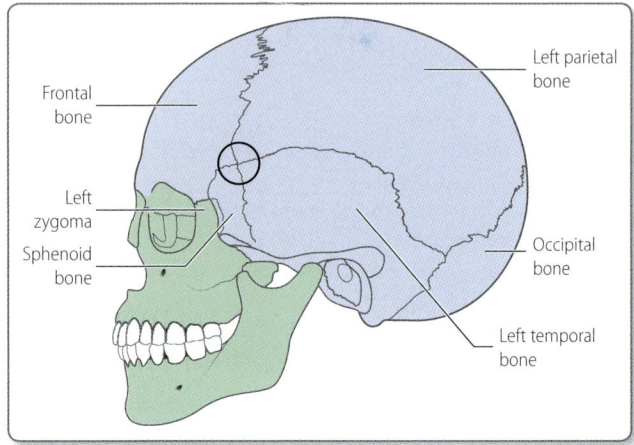

Figure 1.1 Left lateral view of the skull. The neurocranium is shown in blue, and the splanchnocranium in green. The pterion (circled) is the region where the frontal, parietal, temporal and sphenoid bones meet.

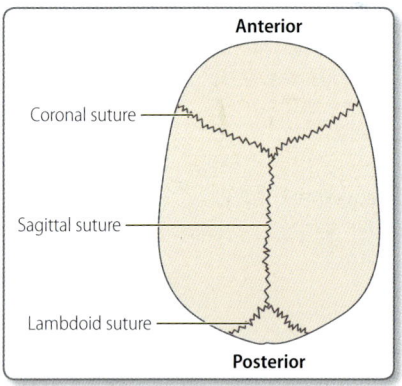

Figure 1.2 Superior view of the coronal, sagittal and lambdoid sutures.

The skull vault The skull vault (also called the calvaria) comprises the frontal, parietal (left and right), occipital, temporal (left and right), sphenoid and ethmoid bones (**Figure 1.1**). In the fully developed skull, these bones are strongly held together by fibrous joints called sutures, such as the sagittal, coronal and lambdoid sutures on the superior aspect (**Figure 1.2**).

The skull base

This anatomically complex structure forms the floor of the cranial cavity. It has many foramina, through which the spinal cord, cranial nerves, blood vessels and other structures pass in or out of the cavity. The largest of the foramina is the foramen magnum.

The skull base is divided into the three cranial fossae: anterior, middle and posterior (**Figure 1.3**). The small hypophyseal fossa, located in the middle fossa, holds the pituitary gland.

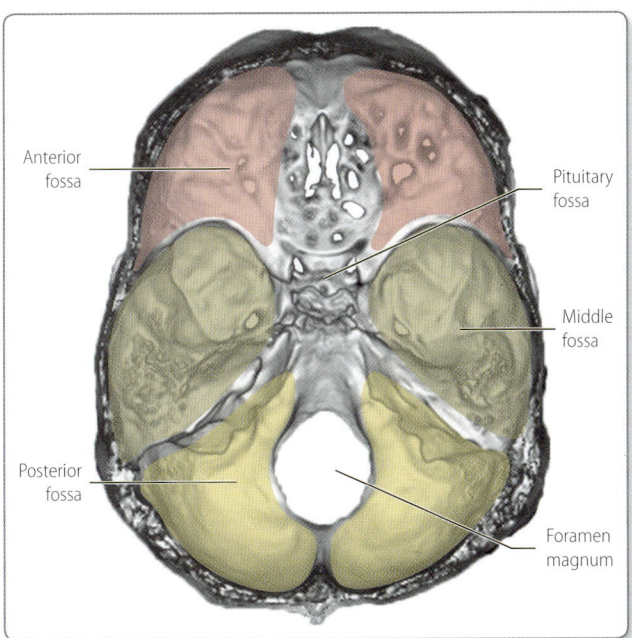

Figure 1.3 Superior view of the anterior, middle and posterior fossae of the skull base.

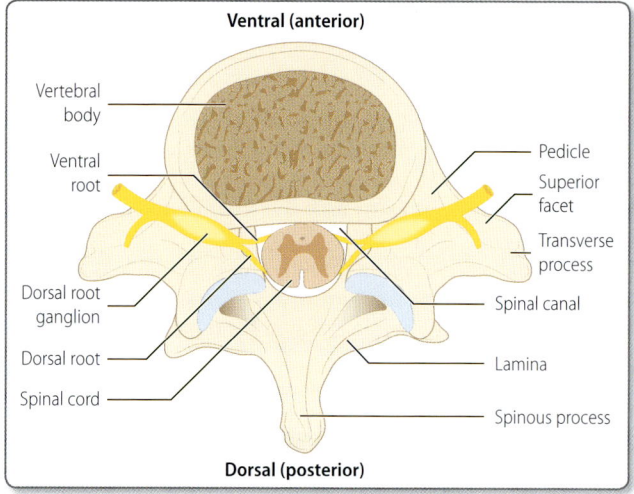

Figure 1.4 A typical vertebra and its relationship to the spinal cord and nerve roots.

The spine

The spine protects the spinal cord. It is a column of individual bones called vertebrae; these differ in structure according to their level but have several key features in common, as shown in **Figure 1.4**. From superior to inferior, the vertebrae are (**Figure 1.5**):

- Seven cervical (C1 to C7)
- Twelve thoracic (T1 to T12)
- Five lumbar (L1 to L5)
- Five sacral (S1 to S5)
- Four coccygeal (Co1 to Co4; these are fused together)

The vertebral bodies are separated by intervertebral discs. Each disc consists of an inner nucleus pulposus and an outer annulus fibrosis.

The cervical spine has several distinct features (**Figure 1.6**), including:

- The first cervical vertebra (C1) is called the atlas; it forms a joint with the occipital condyles (the atlanto-occipital joint)

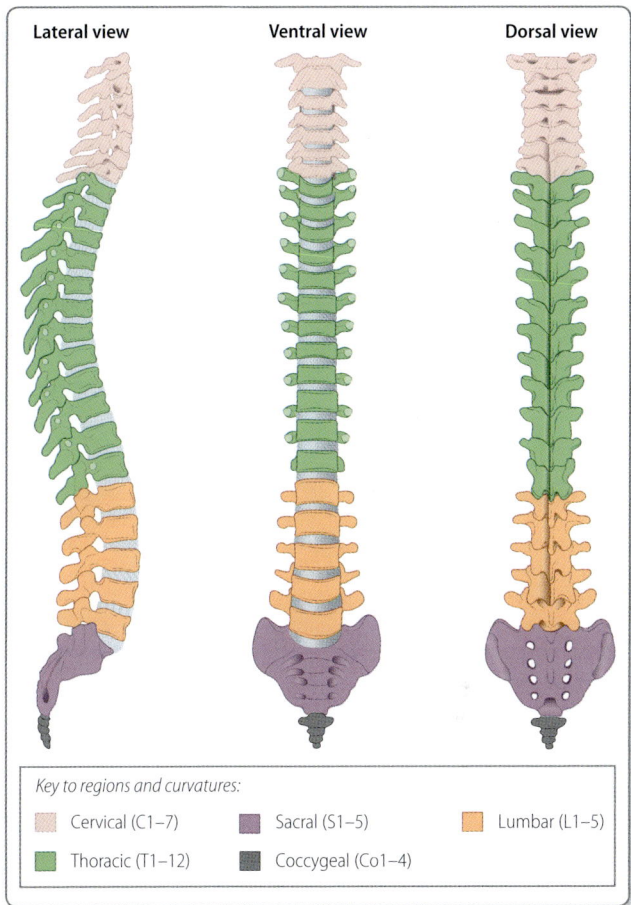

| Lateral view | Ventral view | Dorsal view |

Key to regions and curvatures:

Cervical (C1–7)   Sacral (S1–5)   Lumbar (L1–5)

Thoracic (T1–12)   Coccygeal (Co1–4)

Figure 1.5 Lateral, ventral and dorsal views of the spine, showing the cervical, thoracic, lumbar, sacral and coccygeal divisions.

- The second cervical vertebra (C2) is called the axis; its odontoid process forms a pivot joint with the atlas to allow rotation of the head
- All but the seventh vertebral body of the cervical spine have transverse foramina, which transmit the vertebral arteries

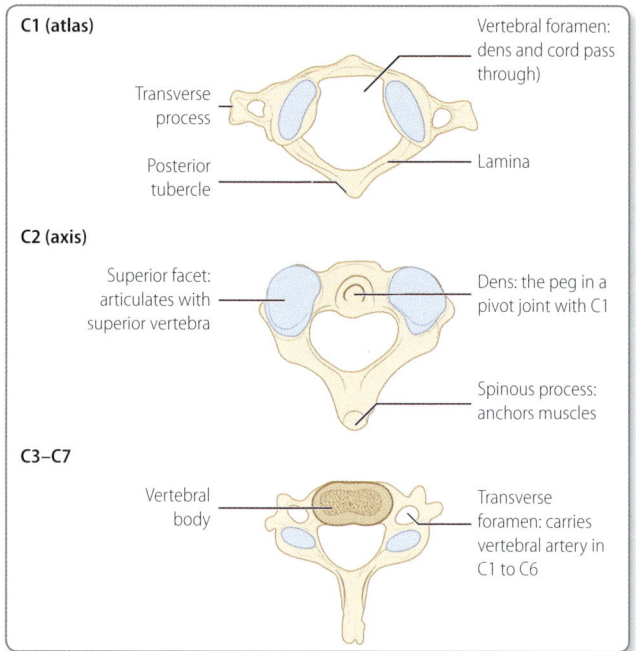

C1 (atlas)

Transverse process

Posterior tubercle

Vertebral foramen: dens and cord pass through)

Lamina

C2 (axis)

Superior facet: articulates with superior vertebra

Dens: the peg in a pivot joint with C1

Spinous process: anchors muscles

C3–C7

Vertebral body

Transverse foramen: carries vertebral artery in C1 to C6

Figure 1.6 Features of the cervical vertebrae.

The meninges

The brain is separated from the skull by three membranous layers called the meninges: the dura, arachnoid and pia mater (**Figure 1.7**). The meninges extend down the spinal canal to encompass the spinal cord, cauda equina and nerve roots. The dura and arachnoid mater terminates at S2, but an extension of the pia mater, the filum terminale, continues to the coccyx.

Dura mater

The dura mater is the thick, outermost layer of the meninges, and itself has an outer (periosteal) and an inner (meningeal) layer. The outer layer of the dura mater is largely adherent to

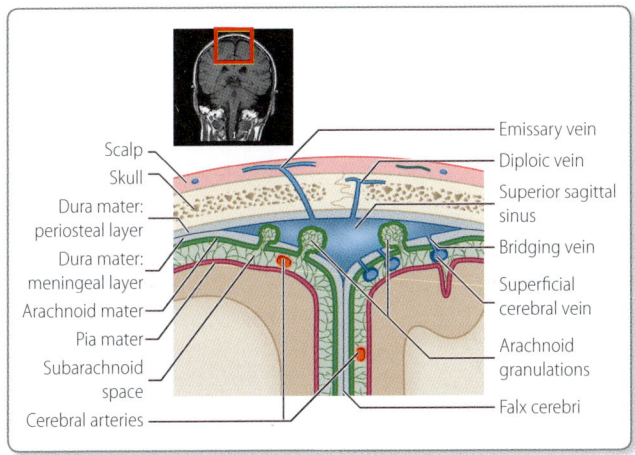

Figure 1.7 The scalp, skull and meninges.

the skull. The inner layer deviates deeply at two main locations to form the falx cerebri (within the longitudinal fissure, which separates the right and left cerebral hemispheres) and the tentorium cerebelli (which separates the cerebrum from the cerebellum). The dural venous sinuses are the channels formed between the separation of the two dural layers.

Arachnoid mater
Deep to the dura mater is the arachnoid mater. The arachnoid mater is in contact with the dura mater but separated from the pia mater by the subarachnoid space. Within the subarachnoid space are cerebral arteries, and veins that drain into the dural venous sinuses via bridging veins. Large subarachnoid spaces are termed cisterns.

Pia mater
The pia mater is the innermost meningeal layer. It is in contact with the surface of the brain.

The cerebrum

The cerebrum is divided into two hemispheres, left and right, separated by the longitudinal (or interhemispheric) fissure. The hemispheres are subdivided into lobes: frontal, temporal, parietal and occipital (**Figure 1.8**). Each lobe has specific functions (**Table 1.1**).

Guiding principle

The functions of the left and right hemispheres are not identical. Areas responsible for language processing (Wernicke's area and Broca's area) are typically located within the dominant hemisphere. This is the left hemisphere in most people, regardless of whether they are right- or left-handed. Therefore, left hemisphere lesions involving the language areas (e.g. stroke or tumour) cause language deficits.

Cerebral cortex

The cerebral cortex is the superficial layer of the brain. It has a convoluted structure characterised by gyri and sulci. Two of the most prominent sulci are the central sulcus (or Rolandic fissure), which divides the frontal and parietal lobes, and the lateral sulcus

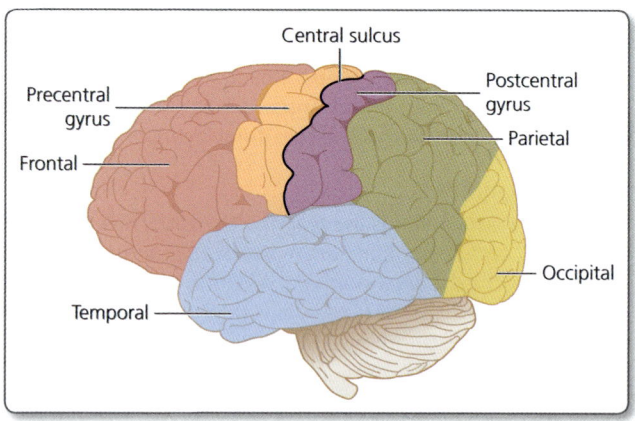

Figure 1.8 Lobes of the brain. The postcentral gyrus (somatosensory region) is part of the parietal lobe. The precentral gyrus (primary motor cortex) is part of the frontal lobe.

Lobe	Function(s)
Frontal	Voluntary movement (primary motor cortex)
	Language* (Broca's area)
	Emotion and personality
	Intelligence and problem-solving
	Attention
Temporal	Language* (Wernicke's area)
	Hearing (auditory area)
	Memory
Parietal	Sensation (somatosensory cortex)
	Spatial orientation †
	Processing and integration of sensory information
Occipital	Vision

*Functions of the dominant hemisphere.
†Functions of the non-dominant hemisphere.

Table 1.1 Key functions of the cerebrum according to lobe

(or Sylvian fissure), which separates the frontal and temporal lobes. The cortex is made up of grey matter, which consists of neuronal cell bodies.

Subcortical structures

White matter is located within the inner part of the cerebrum. It is composed of neuronal axons surrounded by myelin (accounting for the white appearance). Arranged in bundles, these axons form tracts connecting regions of the brain and spinal cord. The corpus callosum is a large white matter tract that connects the two hemispheres of the cerebrum.

Other important subcortical structures include (**Figure 1.9**):

The basal ganglia This is a group of interconnected subcortical nuclei including the subthalamic nucleus, putamen, caudate nucleus and globus pallidus. They act as a circuit to help fine-tune voluntary movements.

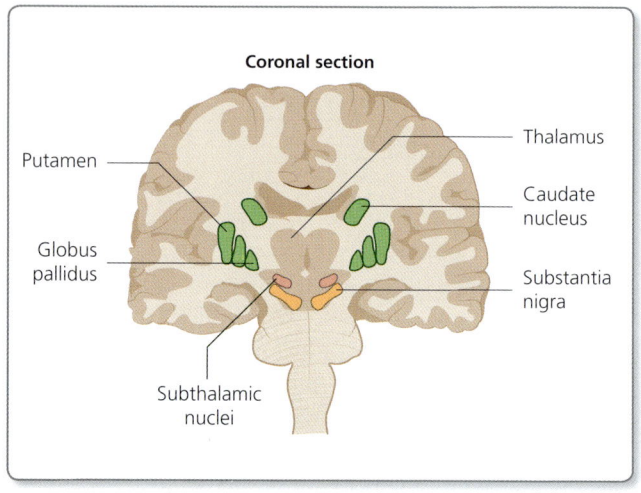

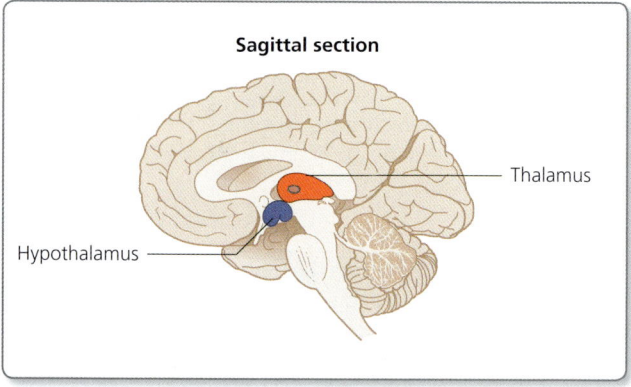

Figure 1.9 Coronal and sagittal sections through the deep structures of the brain.

The internal capsule This is a pathway for the white matter tracts ascending to or descending from the cerebral cortex.

The thalamus The thalamus relays motor and sensory information to and from the cerebral cortex. It also has a key role in the regulation of consciousness.

The hypothalamus This is located inferior to the thalamus and superior to the pituitary gland. Its functions include mediation of emotional responses and maintenance of homeostasis (e.g. body temperature and blood pressure). The hypothalamus influences the autonomic nervous system and the release of hormones from the pituitary gland.

> **Clinical insight**
>
> The proximity of the pituitary gland to the optic chiasm means that a space-occupying lesion of the pituitary gland may cause bitemporal hemianopia (loss of peripheral vision).

The pituitary gland

Connected to the hypothalamus by the stalk-like infundibulum, the pituitary gland lies inferior to the optic chiasm (the point at which fibres from the left and right optic nerves cross) (**Figure 1.10**), and sits within the hypophyseal fossa in the middle cranial fossa. It is divided into an anterior and a posterior lobe. As the so-called 'master gland', it controls the secretion of hormones from other endocrine glands.

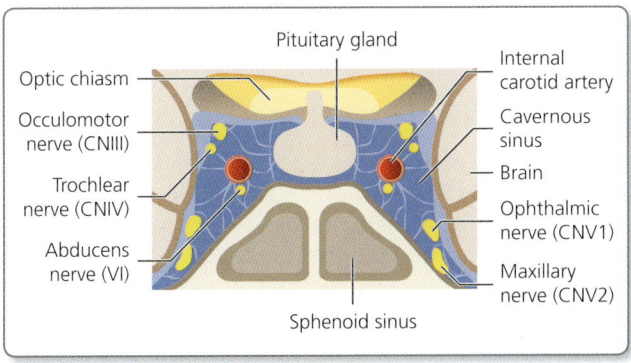

Figure 1.10 Coronal section of the pituitary gland and surrounding anatomy.

The cerebellum

The cerebellum lies in the posterior fossa. It is connected to the brainstem by the superior, middle and inferior cerebellar peduncles.

It has a complex array of folds, called folia, and is divided into the following (**Figure 1.11**):

- The left and right hemispheres, divided by the midline vermis
- The anterior and posterior lobes, divided by the primary fissure

The cerebellum coordinates movement.

The brainstem

The brainstem is divided into three structures (**Figure 1.12**). From superior to inferior, these are the:

- Midbrain
- Pons
- Medulla

The brainstem is responsible for regulation several vital functions, including:

- the respiratory and cardiovascular systems
- the sleep–wake cycle
- arousal and consciousness
- bowel and bladder control
- nausea and vomiting
- pain

It is also where the nuclei of the cranial nerves (III to XII) are located. Running through the brainstem are white matter tracts made up of the axons of motor and sensory pathways, which enable communication between the brain and the spinal cord.

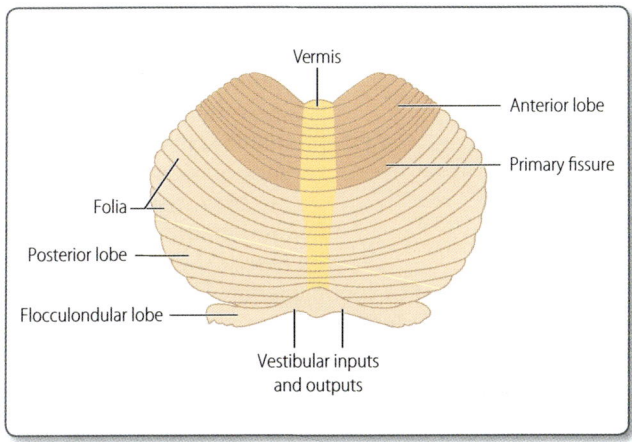

Figure 1.11 The cerebellum: anterior lobe, posterior lobe, vermis, primary fissure, folia.

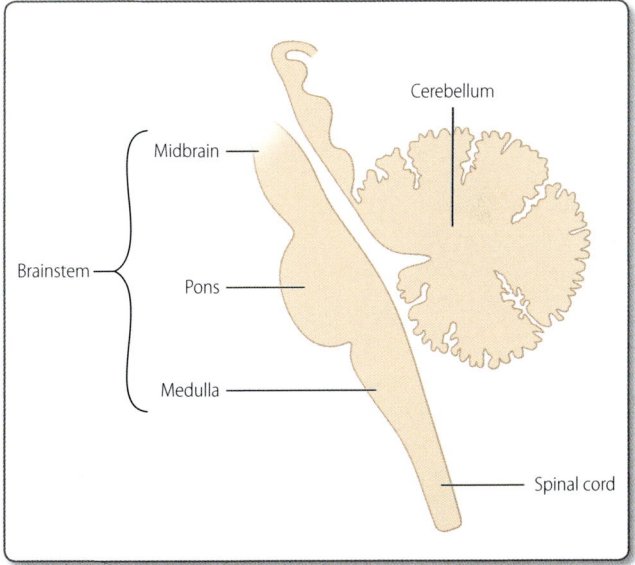

Figure 1.12 The brainstem.

Clinical insight

Most of the fibres of the corticospinal tract decussate (cross from one side of the midline to the other) at the medullary pyramids. This explains why a lesion (e.g. a stroke or tumour) involving the right corticospinal tract above the medulla causes left-sided weakness.

The spinal cord

The spinal cord is contained within the spinal canal, the space formed by the vertebral foramina of successive vertebrae. It extends from the brainstem via the foramen magnum in the skull base, to the conus medullaris at about the level of L1 (normal range, T12 to L2). From the conus medullaris, the lumbar and sacral nerve roots descend

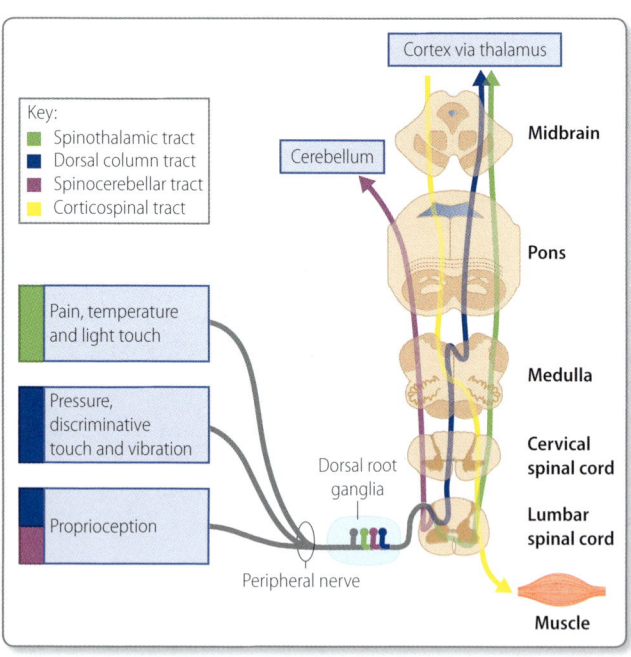

Figure 1.13 The ascending (sensory) and descending (motor) spinal tracts.

unbound; the extending nerve roots are known collectively as the cauda equina.

The spinal cord gives rise to 31 pairs of spinal nerves. The cervical spine has seven vertebrae and the cord has eight cervical spinal nerves:

- each pair of the C1–C7 nerve roots emerges above the numerically corresponding vertebra, and
- the pair of C8 nerve roots emerges below the C7 vertebra

All subsequent nerve roots arise below their corresponding vertebrae.

The spinal tracts

The spinal cord contains white matter tracts that transmit information either from the brain to the peripheral nerves or vice versa (**Figure 1.13**).

Motor information is transmitted via descending pathways, and sensory information via ascending pathways.

The corticospinal tract This is the pathway of neurones descending from the cortex to synapse with the lower motor neurones. They control voluntary muscle action.

The dorsal (posterior) column This pathway of neurones connects sensory nerve endings to the somatosensory region of the cerebral cortex. It is responsible for conscious proprioception and the sensation of vibration and discriminative touch.

The spinothalamic tract This is the neuronal pathway connecting sensory nerve endings to the somatosensory region of the cerebral cortex. It is responsible for the sensation of crude touch, pain and temperature.

The spinocerebellar tract This pathway of neurones connects sensory nerve endings to the cerebellum. It confers unconscious proprioception.

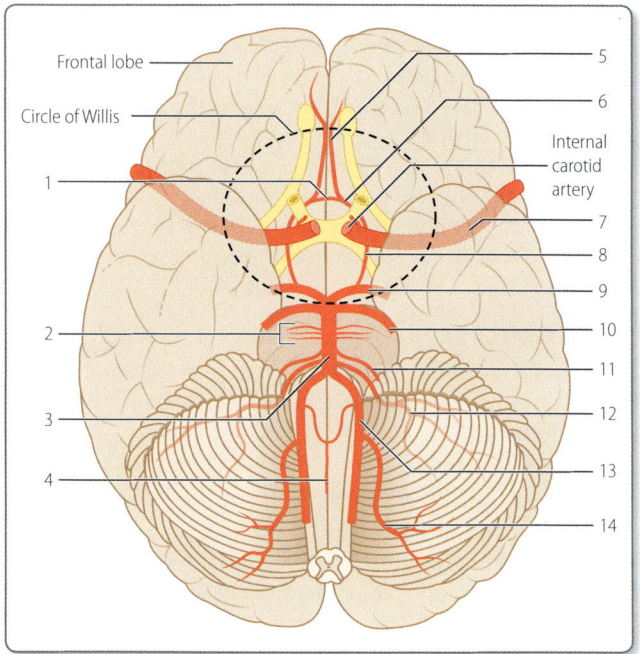

Figure 1.14 The circle of Willis. Key to labels:

① Anterior communicating artery
② Pontine arteries
③ Basilar artery
④ Anterior spinal artery
⑤ Second part (A2) of anterior cerebral artery
⑥ First part (A1) of anterior cerebral artery
⑦ Middle cerebral artery
⑧ Posterior communicating artery
⑨ Posterior cerebral artery
⑩ Superior cerebellar artery
⑪ Labyrinthine artery
⑫ Anterior inferior cerebellar artery
⑬ Vertebral artery
⑭ Posterior inferior cerebellar artery.

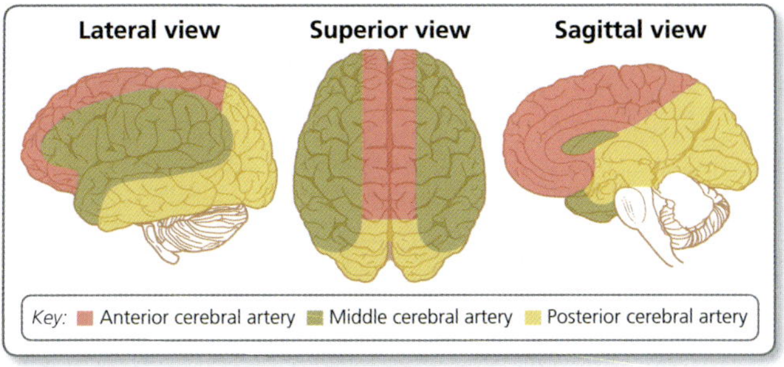

Figure 1.15 Vascular territories of the cerebrum.

The arterial system

Arterial supply to the brain is divided into the anterior circulation and the posterior circulation. The internal carotid and vertebral arteries meet to form an anastomotic structure named the Circle of Willis (**Figure 1.14**), which enables some compensation between the two circulations.

Anterior circulation

The anterior circulation is supplied by the internal carotid arteries. It is the primary supply to the anterior and middle cerebral arteries. The anterior cerebral artery supplies the anteromedial side of the brain (**Figure 1.15**). The middle cerebral artery supplies the lateral side of the brain. The middle cerebral artery gives rise to the lenticulostriate arteries, which supply subcortical structures of the brain (e.g. the basal ganglia).

Posterior circulation

The posterior circulation is supplied by the vertebral arteries. It is the primary supply to the posterior cerebral arteries and the arteries that supply the cerebellum and brainstem. The posterior cerebral arteries supply the base of the cerebrum and the occipital lobes.

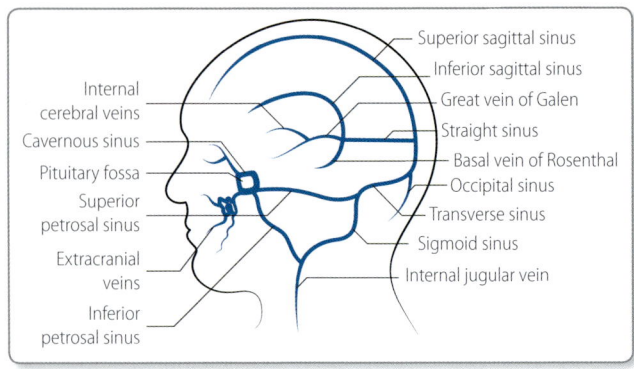

Figure 1.16 Venous drainage of the brain and skull.

The venous system

Cortical veins drain into the dural venous sinuses. The largest sinus is the superior sagittal sinus. Where the major sinuses merge (the confluence of sinuses), the venous blood drains into the left and right transverse sinuses and the left and right sigmoid sinuses, and then the left and right internal jugular veins, respectively (**Figure 1.16**).

The ventricular system

The ventricular system is a collection of four connected compartments filled with cerebrospinal fluid (**Figure 1.17**). The fluid is produced by the specialised tissue of the choroid plexuses, primarily in the lateral ventricles. It flows from the left and right lateral ventricles, via the interventricular foramina (foramina of Munro), to the third ventricle. It then passes through the cerebral aqueduct (aqueduct of Sylvius) to the fourth ventricle. From the fourth ventricle, the fluid either flows into the subarachnoid space, via the median and lateral apertures (foramina of Magendie and Luschka, respectively), before being absorbed by arachnoid granulations into the bloodstream, or flows down through the spinal subarachnoid space or central canal.

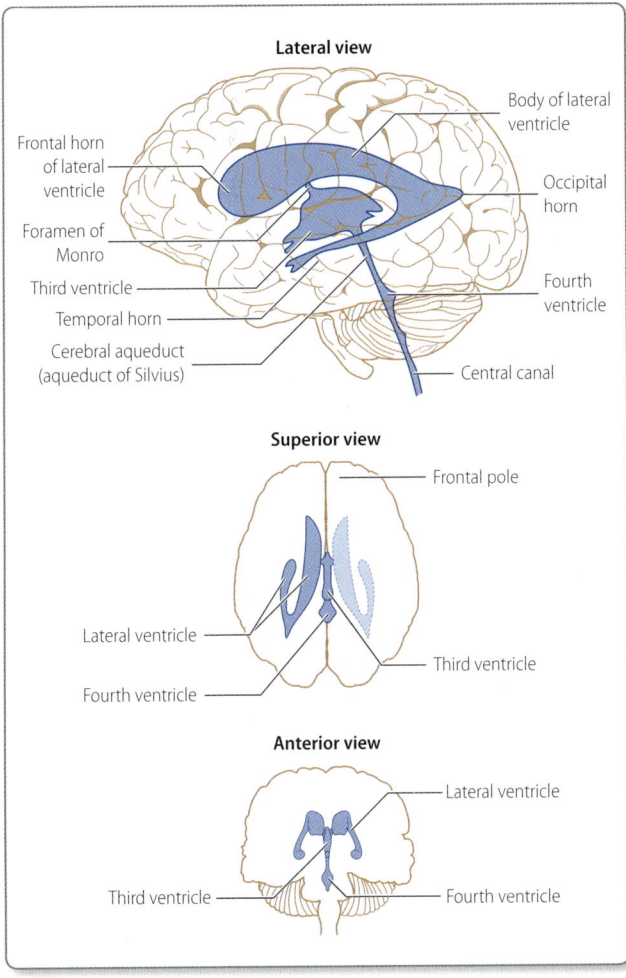

Figure 1.17 Lateral, superior and anterior views of the ventricular system of the brain.

1.2 Radiological terminology

An understanding of the principles of orientation, views and sections is essential to the interpretation of imaging studies. The terms that describe these principles form the language of radiology.

Orientation

The terms used in radiology generally follow those used in anatomy (**Figure 1.18**).

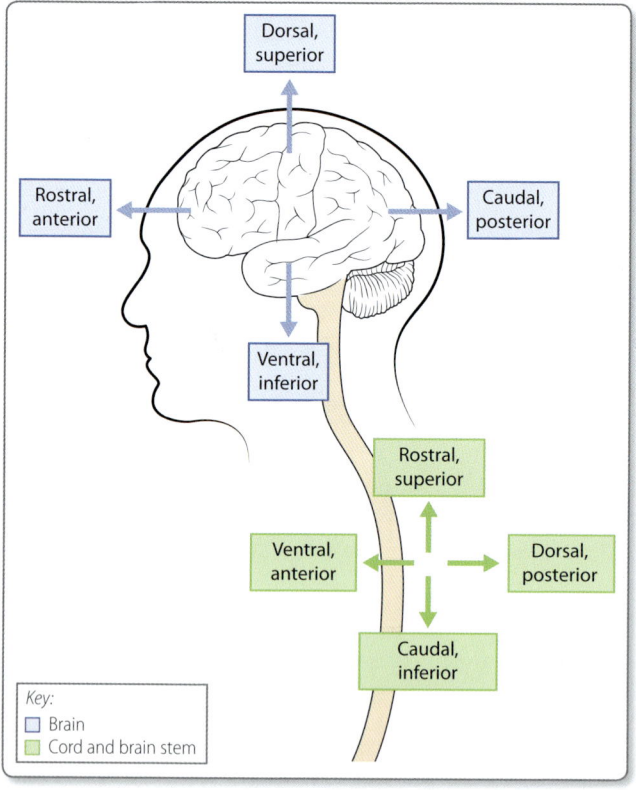

Figure 1.18 Terms used to describe features of the brain and spinal cord.

- **Superior** is used to describe a structure that is higher in position, or situated nearer the top of the head, relative to another structure
- **Inferior** is used to describe a structure that is lower in position, or situated nearer the soles of the feet, relative to another structure
- **Anterior** refers to a structure that is in front of another
- **Posterior** refers to a structure that is behind another
- **Medial** refers to a structure that is closer to the midline of the body relative to another
- **Lateral** refers to a structure that is further away from the midline of the body relative to another
- **Ipsilateral** means on the same side of the body relative to another structure
- **Contralateral** means on the opposite side of the body relative to another structure

These terms are all used consistently in descriptions of features of the brain and spinal cord. In contrast, the terms rostral, caudal, dorsal and ventral have different meanings when applied to features of these two anatomical sites (**Figure 1.18**).

Views

Radiographs are produced by transmitting X-rays through the subject. The direction of transmission determines the view obtained (**Figure 1.19**). An anteroposterior view is produced by transmitting X-rays through the front of the subject towards a detector positioned behind them. A lateral view is produced by transmitting X-rays through the subject from one side (either left or right) towards a detector on the opposite side.

> ### Clinical insight
>
> In CT and MRI, an axial section shows the appearance of internal structures as if viewed from the patient's feet through towards their head. Therefore, the left side of the image corresponds to the right side of the patient.

Sections

In modern neuroimaging (computerised tomography, CT, and magnetic resonance imaging, MRI), multiplanar techniques are

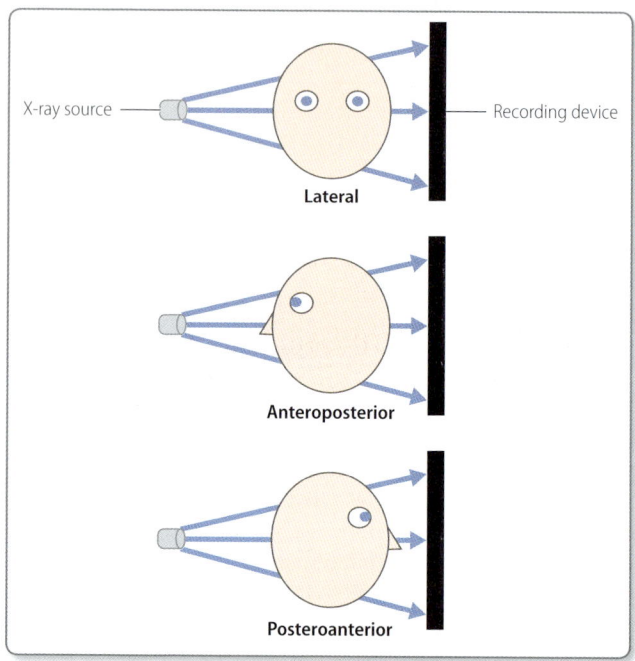

Figure 1.19 Principles of radiographic image acquisition.

used to visualise the brain and spinal cord in cross-sections, or 'slices' (**Figure 1.20**).

- A **sagittal** section provides an image of the brain or spinal cord in a lateral plane (i.e. from the side), which shows relations between structures in terms of superior versus inferior and anterior versus posterior
- An **axial** (or **transverse**) section provides an image of the brain or spinal cord in a horizontal plane, enabling comparison of anterior versus posterior and medial versus lateral structures
- A **coronal** section provides an image of the brain or spinal cord between a front portion and a back portion (similar to an anteroposterior view in radiography); it shows relations between superior versus inferior and medial versus lateral structures

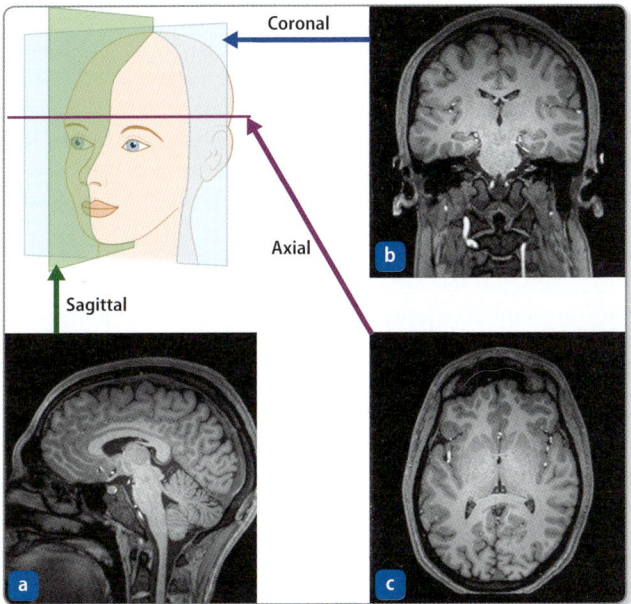

Figure 1.20 T1-weighted MRI scan of the head, showing sagittal (a), coronal (b) and axial (c) sections.

1.3 Imaging modalities

A basic understanding of the principles underlying different neuroimaging modalities facilitates interpretation of the images obtained.

Plain radiography

Radiographs are generally easy to acquire (even possible at the bedside), widely available, rapidly acquired, cost effective and have a significantly lower radiation dose than CT. Due to advances in multi-planar neuroimaging, CT and MRI have largely superseded plain radiography in neuroimaging.

Principles

X-rays from a single-source radiation emitter are directed at the body part of interest, positioned in front of an X-ray detector (film or digital). The X-rays are attenuated (absorbed or scattered) to varying degrees by body tissues of different densities. The resulting variation in X-rays reaching the detector is visualised as differences in contrast in the image captured, i.e. the radiograph.

Applications

In a radiograph, it is not possible to differentiate the skull from the intracranial contents, because X-rays are highly attenuated by the skull. Therefore, radiography is not used for imaging studies of the brain. However, there are specific indications for skull radiographs in clinical practice, for example to visualise the characteristic lytic lesions of multiple myeloma, for ventriculoperitoneal shunt series, and for skeletal surveys in non-accidental injury in children.

Plain radiographs are routinely used to image the spinal column. Indications include trauma (to investigate for fractures, vertebral alignment and stability), spinal deformities (e.g. scoliosis), degeneration and spinal column tumours. Similarly to skull radiographs, the spinal cord cannot be visualised on spine radiographs due to the high density of the spinal column.

Computerised tomography

The availability and fast image acquisition of CT makes it the imaging modality of choice in neurological emergencies (such as trauma and acute cerebrovascular conditions). The advantages and limitations of CT compared with those of MRI are shown in **Table 1.2**.

> ## Clinical insight
>
> Digital subtraction angiography is a fluoroscopy technique (an adaptation of radiography) in which an image intensifier and contrast agents are used to generate real-time images of the intracranial vasculature. It is used in diagnostic and therapeutic interventional neuroradiology procedures.

Principles

Computerised tomography images the body in cross-section. This is an advantage over plain radiography, in which the interpretation of

Feature	CT	MRI
Advantages	Rapid acquisition of images (seconds) Superior detail in images of bone (skull and spine)	No ionising radiation Superior detail in images of soft tissues Superior detail in images of brain and spinal cord
Limitations	Ionising radiation	Slow acquisition (minutes) Difficult for paediatric patients (anaesthesia often required) Susceptibility to motion artefact Claustrophobia Noise Magnetic risks and incompatibility issues (e.g. pacemaker)

Table 1.2 Comparison of computerised tomography (CT) and magnetic resonance imaging (MRI)

images is made difficult by the superimposition of body tissues of different densities.

Beams of X-rays are directed through the patient along multiple linear paths and measured by a series of X-ray detectors (**Figure 1.21**). Attenuation values for each discrete three-dimensional element of volume (voxel; **Figure 1.22**) is calculated using data from X-ray paths intersecting at the coordinates of the voxel. Using these values, a three-dimensional density map can be visualised as grey-scale image that we can interpret.

Applications

The introduction of contrast agents into the vascular system significantly increases the density of blood vessels, thereby enabling them to be clearly differentiated from surrounding body tissue. Usually the contrast agent is an iodinated compound because their density is clearly visible on CT, they are soluble and do not harm the body. Contrast is used in CT angiography, CT venography and also to identify dysfunction of the blood–brain barrier (e.g. in the case of contrast-enhancing brain tumours).

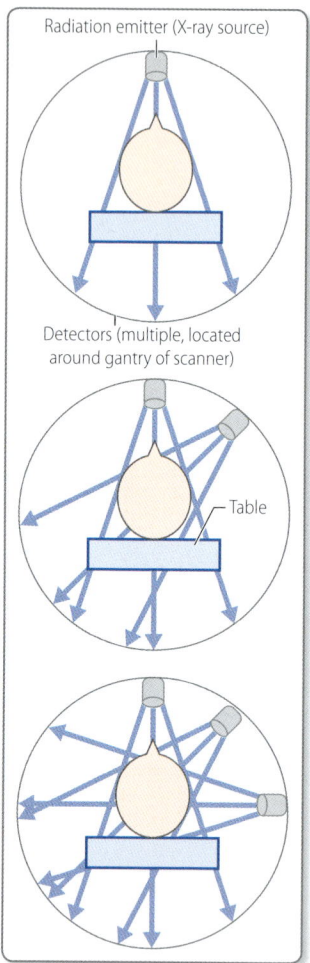

Radiation emitter (X-ray source)

Detectors (multiple, located around gantry of scanner)

Table

Figure 1.21 CT image acquisition. In plain radiography, a single X-ray beam is transmitted through the patient towards a detector. In CT, the X-ray emitters and detectors rotate around the scanner gantry in order to transmit X-rays in multiple, intersecting paths. Using a method called 'back-projection', the attenuation at each voxel is calculated.

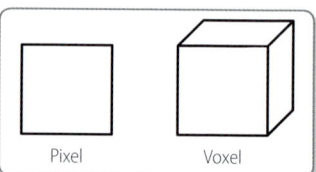

Pixel   Voxel

Figure 1.22 A pixel (a picture element) is two-dimensional, i.e. is a square. A voxel (a volume element) is three-dimensional, i.e. is a cube or cuboid.

CT angiography Contrast is used to improve visualisation of the arterial system. In the context of neuroimaging, it is used to identify vascular abnormalities such as aneurysms.

CT venography Contrast is also used to improve visualisation of the venous system. The venous system can be enhanced selectively by increasing the delay between contrast administration and image acquisition. This technique can be used to investigate for dural venous sinus thrombosis.

CT perfusion This measures cerebral blood flow. It is used to determine the amount of salvageable parenchyma (the penumbra) in patients who have had a stroke, and to identify vasospasm in subarachnoid haemorrhage.

Magnetic resonance imaging

Magnetic resonance imaging (MRI) is a powerful neuroimaging modality. It shows both the structures and pathology of the brain and spinal cord in better detail than CT. However, image acquisition is much longer, the scanner is more claustrophobic and patients can be upset by the loud noises that it makes. **Table 1.2** compares the advantages and limitations of MRI and CT.

Principles

MRI is based on altering the properties of the abundant hydrogen atoms within the body. This is done by exposing the patient to the strong magnetic field of the large cylindrical magnet that is part of the MRI scanner (**Figure 1.23**).

Each hydrogen atom contains a single proton nucleus that spins around a central axis. In the magnetic field of the MRI scanner, the central axis of each proton aligns with the direction of the magnetic field. Although aligned, the protons spin out of phase with each other. A radiofrequency pulse is then applied, which causes the central axis of each proton to realign perpendicular to the direction of the magnetic field; consequently, all the protons spin in phase. When the radiofrequency pulse ceases, each proton's central axis realigns with the direction of the magnetic field, and the protons gradually return to spinning out of phase.

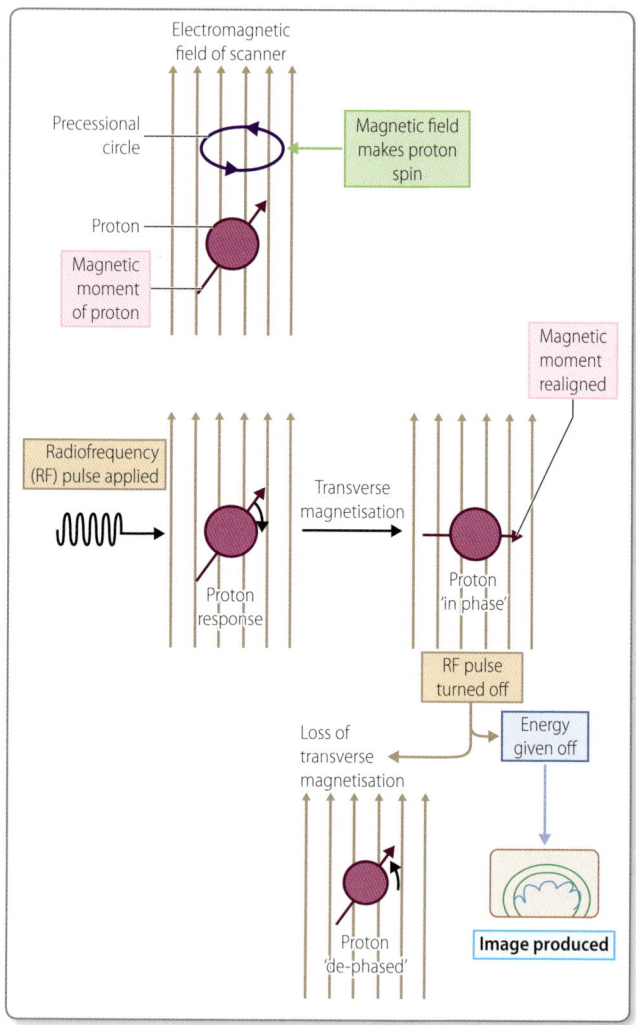

Figure 1.23 MRI image acquisition.

Variation in both the alignment of the protons and their phase of spin results in different signals for different tissues. This is represented by differences in the greyscale image generated.

Clinical MRI scanners vary in the strength of their magnetic field (for which the unit is the tesla, T); strengths of 1.5 and 3.0 T are typical. The higher the number of teslas, the higher the signal-to-noise ratio.

Applications

Contrast agents are used in MRI to enhance imaging of blood–brain barrier disruption, tumours, inflammation, demyelination and infection. Gadolinium is a commonly used contrast agent used in MRI and works by increasing signal on T1-weighted imaging.

Magnetic resonance angiography and venography These techniques use specific magnetic resonance signals to improve visualisation of the arteries and veins, respectively. Unlike CT angiography and CT venography, they do not necessarily re-quire the use of a contrast agent.

Diffusion-weighted imaging This technique is used to esti-mate the diffusion of water in tissue. It is used to investigate for cerebral ischaemia, infection, traumatic brain injury and degenerative disease.

Diffusion tensor imaging This is used to study the direction of diffusion within tissues, and can be used to determine the orientation of white matter tracts. In tractography (also called fibre-tracking), data from diffusion tensor imaging are used to generate a three-dimensional map of the white matter tracts. Tractography is increasingly being used for neurosurgical plan-ning and intraoperative guidance.

Functional MRI This is used to measure brain activity. It uses the technique of blood oxygenation level–dependent imag-ing to show regions of increased blood flow and oxygenation, which are assumed to represent regions of increased neuronal activity. As well as being an increasingly useful tool in neuropsychological research, functional MRI is used to prevent iatrogenic injury and subsequent post-surgical neurological deficits in patients undergoing neurosurgery.

MRI spectroscopy This technique is used to measure the chemical composition of tissue. Chemicals measured include *N*-acetylaspartate, choline, lactate, creatine and glutamate. Spectroscopy is used to investigate and differentiate between brain lesions (e.g. tumours, infarcts and infections).

MRI perfusion This is similar to CT perfusion. It allows the approximate quantification of cerebral blood flow and blood volume. It is particularly useful in the assessment of tumours, for their differentiation from tumour mimics and the identification of aggressive features for targeted biopsy.

1.4 Patient safety

Neuroimaging is not without risk. For each patient, the risks of image acquisition need to be carefully balanced against the clinical usefulness of the images that will be obtained.

Radiography and CT imaging

Both plain radiography and CT use ionising radiation. Radiation causes cellular and genetic damage, and significant exposure increases the risk of developing cancer. Modern equipment minimises the radiation dose but cannot eliminate it. In particular, children are more radiosensitive than adults and the risks versus benefits should be especially carefully considered. The fetus is especially susceptible to irradiation injury. All girls and women of child-bearing age are asked if there is any possibility that they could be pregnant. In pregnancy, clinicians may choose a different imaging modality, deferring non-urgent imaging or carrying out a risk–benefit analysis specific to the patient.

Investigation	Average recorded effective dose (mSv)
Skull radiograph	0.1
Chest radiograph	0.2
Cervical spine radiograph	0.2
Thoracic spine radiograph	1.0
Lumbar spine radiograph	1.5
Head CT	2
Spine CT	6
Head and neck angiogram	5
Data from Mettler FA Jr, et al. Radiology 2008; 248:254–263.	

Table 1.3 Effective doses of ionising radiation in radiography and computerised tomography (CT)

The effective dose of radiation to which a patient is exposed is measured in Sieverts (Sv); 1 Sv = 1 J/kg. Example doses are given in **Table 1.3**, which illustrates the higher dose of CT compared with a radiograph.

MRI safety

The MRI scanner contains a large superconducting magnet, and patients are exposed to its magnetic field. There is no evidence that exposure to high-strength magnetic fields contributes to any pathological processes. However, ferromagnetic objects are made hazardous by their strong attraction to the powerful magnetic field.

Clinical insight

Some tattoo inks contain metal components, which may cause the patient to experience a burning sensation. However, this rarely causes harm or intolerable discomfort, so the presence of tattoos is not a contraindication for MRI.

Clinical insight

All patients undergoing MRI are required to complete a safety questionnaire and checklist in order to identify contraindications (e.g. internal ferromagnetic objects).

Any external ferromagnetic material that enters the magnetic field is immediately and forcefully propelled towards the bore (centre) of the scanner; this is known as the missile effect. Potential projectiles that could cause injury include oxygen canisters, metal chairs, jewellery, buckles, etc. These must be removed before imaging.

Internal ferromagnetic materials have the potential to be displaced or distorted. Surgical devices, implants (e.g. cochlear implants) and foreign bodies (e.g. metal fragments in the eye). Electronic devices, such as pacemakers, will be damaged. Displacement or dysfunction of these objects will injure or be life-threatening to the patient.

Contrast reactions

All contrast agents have the potential to cause harm. Some may cause contrast-induced nephropathy, therefore the risk and benefits of imaging requiring contrast in patients with renal impairment should be considered carefully. Other risks include immediate or delayed allergic reaction.

Interpreting normal images

Understanding the normal appearance of the brain and spinal cord with different imaging modalities is a prerequisite for interpretation of abnormal findings in disease. This requires experience, studying as many images as possible. It also requires an appreciation of normal anatomical variation.

2.1 Terminology

Each imaging modality has its own terminology (**Table 2.1**).

Plain radiography

Orientation

Different radiographic views are obtained by transmitting X-rays through the patient from different directions. To interpret a radiograph, the viewer needs to know the view. Radiographers routinely add markers to radiographs, such as 'L' (left) or 'R' (right), to guide the viewer.

Appearance

Radiographic features are described in terms of opacity or lucency, depending on whether they appear bright or dark, respectively. Whether a feature is opaque or lucent is determined by the degree to which it attenuates X-rays, which, in turn, depends on its atomic density (**Figure 2.1**).

Imaging modality	Bright features	Dark features
Plain radiography	Opaque	Lucent
CT	Hyperdense (or hyperattenuating)	Hypodense (or hypoattenuating)
MRI	Hyperintense (or high signal)	Hypointense (or low signal)

Table 2.1 Terms describing images obtained with different imaging modalities

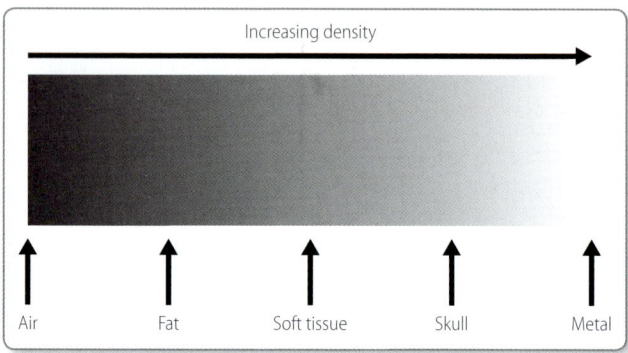

Figure 2.1 X-ray attenuation.

Air has low atomic density, so attenuates very few X-rays; the great majority reach the X-ray detector. This results in the dark radiographic appearance of air. Conversely, bone, which has high atomic density, attenuates X-rays to a far greater degree and therefore appears bright on a radiograph. Fat and soft tissue, which are of intermediate density, are visualised as areas of intermediate brightness.

Skull radiographs are not useful for imaging the brain. The density of the skull is greater than that of the intracranial contents. Therefore, its radiographic opacity precludes visualisation of the brain. Only calcified or other radiographically dense features may be visible.

CT

Orientation

In CT, an axial section presents an image of the brain or spinal cord as if viewed from below, looking towards the top of the patient's head from the soles of their feet (**Figure 2.2a**). This means that the top of the image is anterior, and the left side of the image is the right side of the patient.

A sagittal section presents an image of the brain or spinal cord as if viewed from the side of the patient (**Figure 2.2b**). The right side of the image is conventionally posterior and the top of the image is superior.

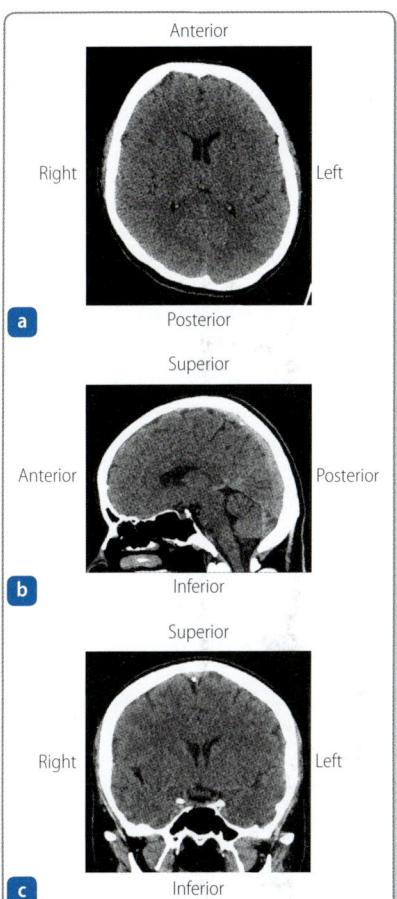

Figure 2.2 Orientation of CT scans. (a) Axial, (b) sagittal and (c) coronal sections.

A coronal section presents an image of the brain or spinal cord as if viewed from the front (**Figure 2.2c**). Therefore, the left side of the image is the right side of the patient.

Appearance

In CT, as in plain radiography, dense structures attenuate more X-rays and therefore appear bright, and less dense structures, which attenuate fewer X-rays, appear dark. Therefore, when describing findings on CT:

- Bright features are termed hyperdense (or hyperattenuating)
- Dark features are termed hypodense (or hypoattenuating)
- Features of equal density are termed isodense

The attenuation of X-rays by different materials is quantified in Hounsfield units (HU). The Hounsfield scale used in CT ranges from −1000 HU to +1000 HU. Values along this scale are represented in the image by shades of grey in a continuum ranging from black to white, respectively. **Figure 2.3** shows the typical distribution of attenuation by air, fat, soft tissue, bone, etc. along the Hounsfield scale.

The range of Hounsfield units represented between absolute black and absolute white on an image, i.e. the 'window', can be changed to manipulate the contrast and thereby improve visualisation of features of interest. The window can be narrowed, widened or moved to a different position along the scale (**Figure 2.4**).

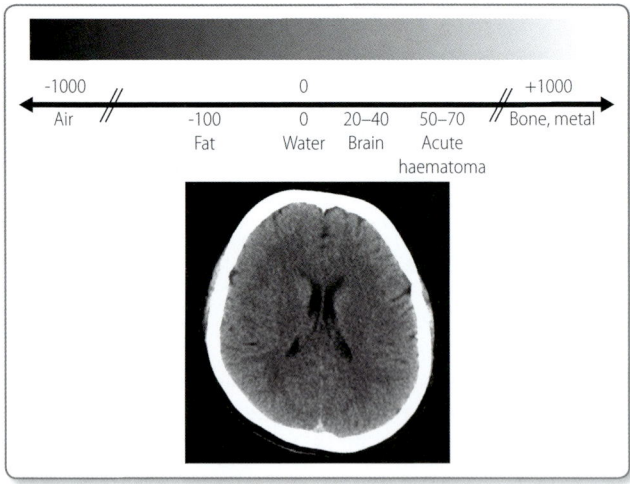

Figure 2.3 The Hounsfield scale used in CT and corresponding neuroimaging correlates.

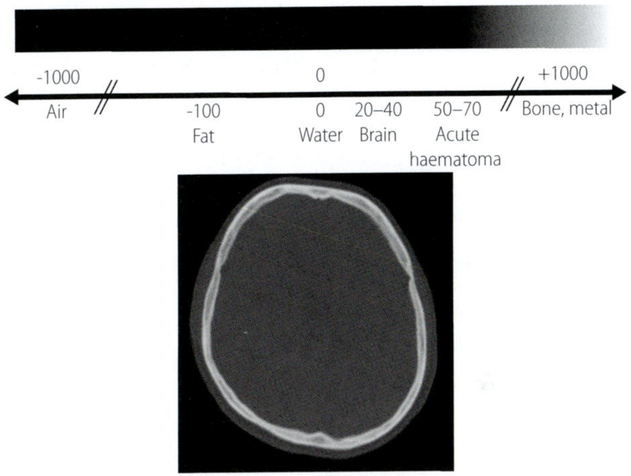

Figure 2.4 Creating a bone window. For the same subject as Figure 2.5, the number of Hounsfield units corresponding to absolute black has been increased (i.e. moved right along the Hounsfield scale). This allows small differences in density to be shown in a greater number of shades of grey, thereby improving visualisation of bone on the CT image.

MRI

Orientation

The general principles of orientation in MRI are the same as those in CT.

Appearance

In MRI, features are described in terms of signal intensity. Bright features are described as 'hyperintense' and dark findings are described as 'hypointense'.

In MRI, different sequences (radiofrequency and pulse settings) are used to improve visualisation of different features. The most commonly used sequences in clinical neuroimaging are T1-weighted, T2-weighted and T2-weighted fluid-attenuated

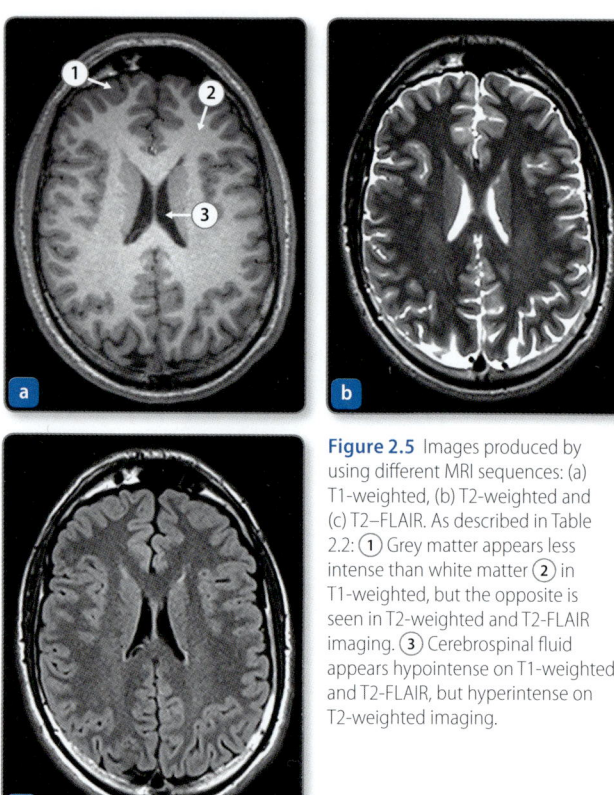

Figure 2.5 Images produced by using different MRI sequences: (a) T1-weighted, (b) T2-weighted and (c) T2–FLAIR. As described in Table 2.2: ① Grey matter appears less intense than white matter ② in T1-weighted, but the opposite is seen in T2-weighted and T2-FLAIR imaging. ③ Cerebrospinal fluid appears hypointense on T1-weighted and T2-FLAIR, but hyperintense on T2-weighted imaging.

inversion recovery (T2–FLAIR) (**Figure 2.5**). The application of these sequences is compared in **Table 2.2**. Several other sequences are used in clinical neuroimaging; in this book, they are described alongside the pathologies for which they are relevant.

	T1-weighted MRI signal	T2-weighted MRI signal
Air	Low	Low
Cortical bone	Low	Low
Soft tissue	Medium	Medium
Grey matter	Lower than that of white matter	Higher than that of white matter
White matter	Higher than that of grey matter	Lower than that of white matter
Cerebrospinal fluid	Low	High
Examples of applications	Anatomy: for differentiation of grey and white matter With contrast enhancement: investigating lesions of brain and spine (e.g. tumour, infection, inflammation)	Inflammation Oedema

Table 2.2 Comparison of T1-weighted and T2-weighted MRI sequences. These are the most utilised sequences in neuroimaging

2.2 Bone: the skull

Plain radiography

Plain radiography has historically been used to visualise the skull to assess fractures, but intracranial pathology (such as a haematoma) cannot be visualised. It has been superseded by CT for this purpose, because CT shows the skull and intracranial appearances in cross sections.

Skull radiographs are indicated when investigating for multiple myeloma ('pepper pot skull') and assessing ventriculoperitoneal shunts. They are also included in skeletal surveys in non-accidental injury in children.

CT

Computerised tomography is the preferred imaging modality for examining bone. It shows the skull in more detail, compared with MRI.

The skull

Use of a bone window enables the skull to be visualised in detail, with a hyperdense inner and outer layer of cortical bone, and a relatively hypodense layer of cancellous bone between these layers (**Figure 2.6**). The sutures are hypodense with saw-toothed hyperdense edges. They should not be mistaken for fracture lines.

The sinuses

The presence of air within the sinuses of the skull means that they normally appear hypodense (**Figure 2.7**). Features of higher density within the sinuses suggest a pathological process, e.g. sinusitis.

The ethmoid air cells and sphenoid sinus communicate with the nasal cavity and are often seen within the same axial section.

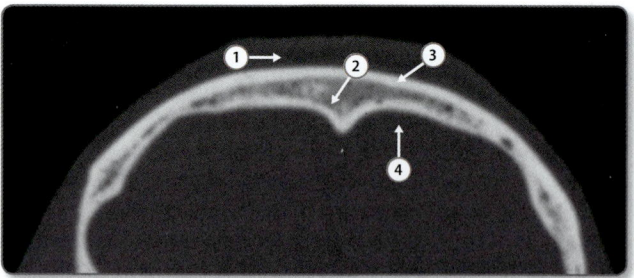

Figure 2.6 Axial CT scan with bone window, showing the frontal bone of the skull. ① The scalp, ② cancellous (medullary) bone, ③ outer cortical bone, ④ inner cortical bone.

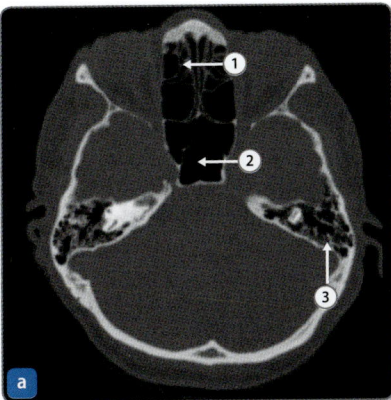

Figure 2.7 CT scan showing sinuses within the skull. ① Ethmoidal air cells, ② sphenoid sinus, ③ mastoid air cells, ④ frontal sinus.

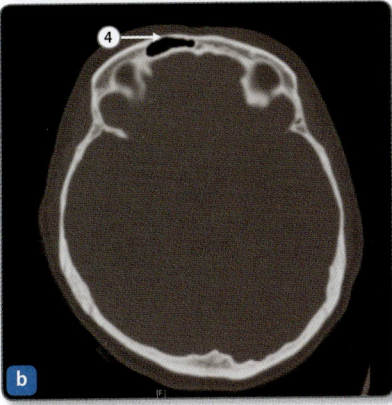

The frontal sinuses are more superior and are within the frontal bone. The maxillary sinuses are more inferior. The mastoid air cells communicate with the middle ear. The sinuses are highly variable in appearance between healthy individuals. They may or may not have several septa.

2.3 Bone: the spine

Plain radiography

Plain radiographs are used in investigations of the spine for vertebral fractures. Similar to plain radiographs of the skull unable to reveal the brain, plain radiographs of the spine are unable to show the structure of the spinal cord due to the high density of the surrounding vertebrae.

The cervical spine

Three views are routinely obtained: lateral (**Figure 2.8**), antero-posterior (**Figure 2.9**) and odontoid (**Figure 2.10**). An odontoid view is obtained by transmission of X-rays in an anterior to posterior direction through the patient's open mouth; this enables visualisation of a prominence of the C2 vertebra called the odontoid process.

The following system can be used to assess cervical spine radiographs.

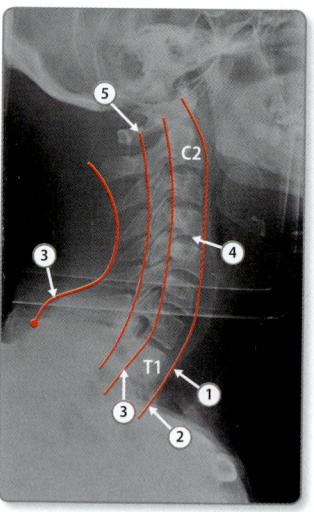

Figure 2.8 Plain radiograph (lateral view) of the cervical spine. ① C7–T1 junction, ② anterior vertebral line, ③ posterior vertebral line, ④ intervertebral disc space ⑤ spinolaminar line.

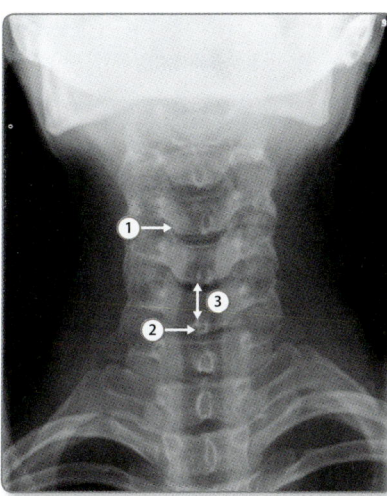

Figure 2.9 Plain radiograph (anteroposterior view) of the cervical spine.
① Uncovertebral joints.
② Spinous processes.
③ Distance between the spinous processes.

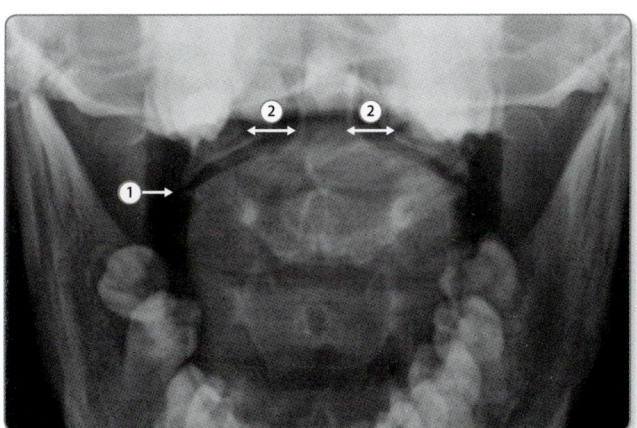

Figure 2.10 Plain radiograph (odontoid view) of the cervical spine. ① Normal alignment of the lateral masses of C1 and C2, ② distance between the odontoid process and the lateral masses of C1.

Lateral view

A lateral view is acquired to assess the alignment, integrity and spacing of the vertebrae.

- The C7–T1 junction must be visible for the radiograph to be considered adequate
- Alignment of the vertebrae is assessed by checking the integrity of the anterior vertebral line, posterior vertebral line, spinolaminar line and posterior spinous line
- The integrity of each vertebral body, the intervertebral disc spaces, the laminae, the facets and the spinous processes is assessed
- The intervertebral disc spaces should be of equal height
- The space between the atlas and the odontoid process (i.e. the atlanto–odontoid distance) should be less than 4 mm
- The normal width of the prevertebral tissue should be less than 7 mm at C1–C4, and less than 22 mm at C5–C7

Anteroposterior view

- Alignment of the vertebral bodies and spinous processes is assessed on an anteroposterior view
- As in the lateral view, the heights of the intervertebral discs should be equal

Odontoid view

- Allows assessment of the articulation of C1 and C2
- The spaces between the odontoid process and each of the lateral masses should be equal

The thoracic and lumbar spine

Lateral and anteroposterior views of the thoracic and lumbar spines are routinely obtained (**Figures 2.11** and **2.12**).

- The adequacy of the radiographs is assessed by ensuring that the entire region (i.e. all the thoracic vertebrae or all the lumbar vertebrae) is visible
- Alignment is assessed by inspecting the anterior and posterior vertebral lines
- The integrity of the vertebral bodies, pedicles and spinous processes is assessed

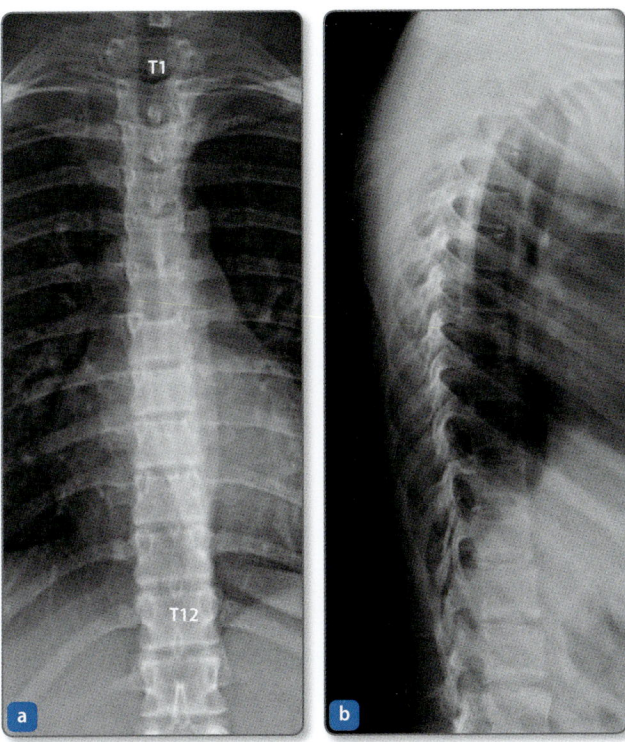

Figure 2.11 Plain radiographs of the thoracic spine: (a) anteroposterior and (b) lateral view.

- Intervertebral disc height and spacing are assessed

CT

The relation between density and greyscale appearance in CT is the same as in plain radiography and MRI. However, unlike plain radiography, CT allows the spine to be viewed in cross-section, and it provides a more detailed view of the spine

Guiding principle

It is difficult to visualise the complex structure of the spine based on images of single CT 'slices' displayed on a page. The three-dimensional structure is better appreciated by scrolling through multiple slices.

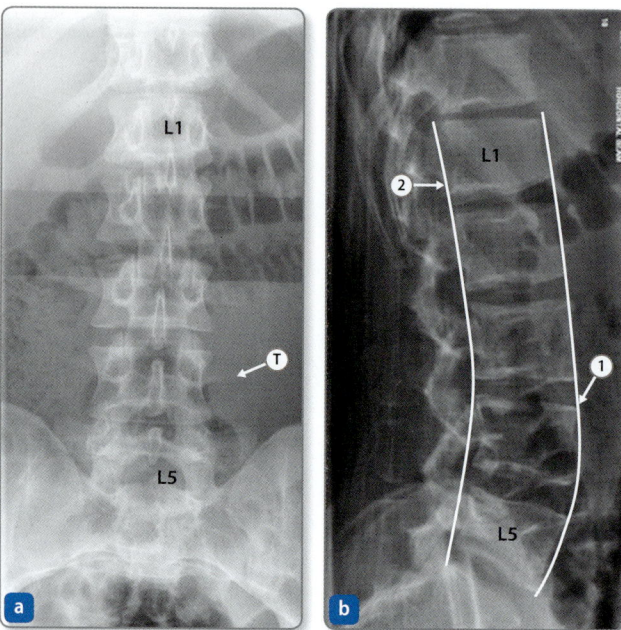

Figure 2.12 Plain radiographs of the lumbar spine: (a) anteroposterior and (b) lateral view. ① Anterior vertebral line, ② posterior vertebral line, Ⓣ transverse processes.

than is possible with MRI. A bone window is used (**Figure 2.13**). Axial, sagittal and coronal sections can be obtained.

2.4 The meninges

CT

The normal meninges are not well visualised on CT. The dura and arachnoid mater are confluent with the skull, and the pia mater is thin and confluent with the brain. However, the two infoldings of dura mater, i.e. the falx cerebri (**Figure 2.14**) and the tentorium cerebelli (**Figure 2.15**), appear as thin hyperdense lines.

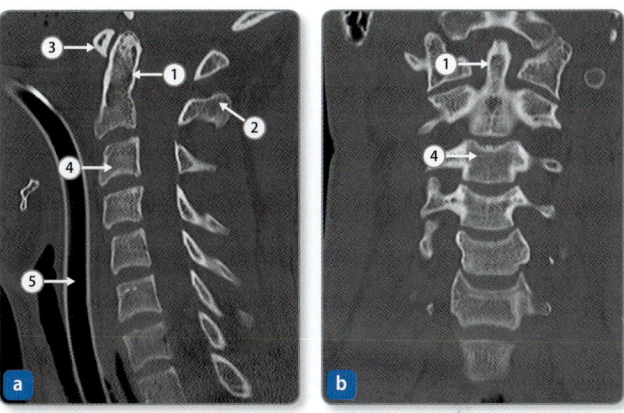

Figure 2.13 CT scans (with bone window) of the cervical spine: (a) sagittal and (b) coronal section. ① Odontoid process, ② spinous processes, ③ anterior arch of C1 (atlas), ④ vertebral body of C3, ⑤ endotracheal tube (the patient was intubated).

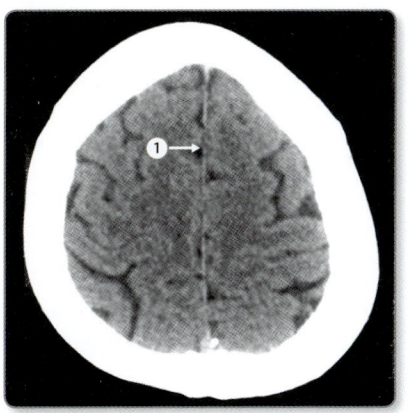

Figure 2.14 Axial CT scan of the head. ① Falx cerebri.

The arachnoid mater is indistinguishable from the dura mater on CT. However, the subarachnoid space (between the arachnoid and pia mater) is hypodense, because it is filled with cerebrospinal fluid.

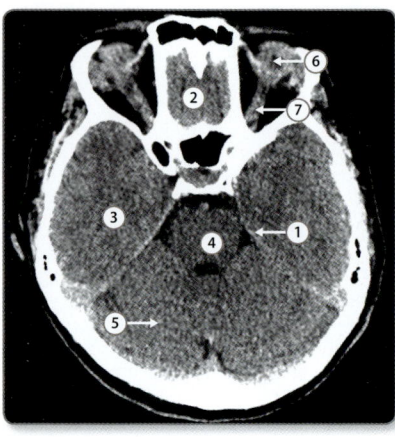

Figure 2.15 Axial CT scan showing the normal brain. ① Tentorium cerebelli, ② frontal lobe, ③ temporal lobe, ④ brainstem, ⑤ cerebellum, ⑥ eye, ⑦ optic nerve.

> ### Clinical insight
>
> Meningitis can be detected on T1-weighted MRI by the presence of leptomeningeal contrast enhancement. This feature represents inflammation of the arachnoid and pia mater.

MRI

The meninges are difficult to visualise on MRI without the use of contrast agent. However, the falx cerebri and tentorium cerebelli appear hyperintense on contrast T1-weighted images.

2.5 The brain

CT

To enable differentiation of the white and grey matter, the range of Hounsfield units is adjusted to accentuate the +20 to +40 HU range. Grey matter, for example that in the cerebral cortex, appears hyperdense compared with white matter (**Figure 2.16**).

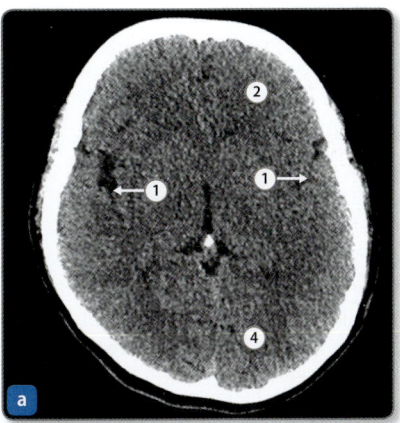

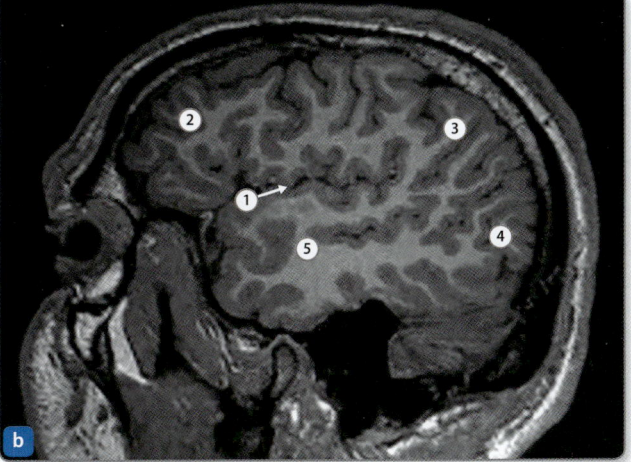

Figure 2.16 (a) Axial CT scan and (b) sagittal T1-weighted MRI scan of the head. ① Lateral sulcus (Sylvian fissure), ② frontal lobe, ③ parietal lobe, ④ occipital lobe, ⑤ temporal lobe.

It is possible to identify the border between the grey matter of the cerebral cortex and the underlying white matter.

MRI

The intensity of grey and white matter on MRI depends on the sequence used (see **Table 2.2**). On T1-weighted images of the adult brain, the white matter is more intense than the grey matter, thus reflecting its appearance in vivo and on CT. On T2-weighted images, however, the white matter is less intense than the grey matter.

Smaller structures within the brain, and finer details, are more easily distinguished on MRI than on CT, because of the superior spatial resolution achieved with MRI. The nuclei of the basal ganglia consist of grey matter and therefore appear relatively hypointense on T1-weighted MRI (**Figure 2.17**) and hyperintense on T2-weighted MRI. Conversely, white matter tracts such as the corpus callosum appear relatively hyperintense on T1-weighted MRI (**Figure 2.18**) and hypointense on T2-weighted MRI.

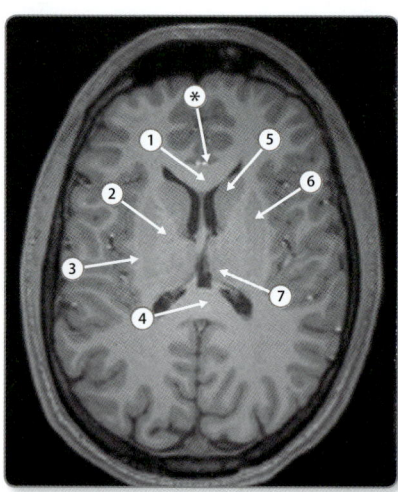

Figure 2.17 Axial T1-weighted MRI scan of the basal ganglia and surrounding subcortical structures. ① Genu of the corpus callosum, ② internal capsule, ③ external capsule, ④ splenium of the corpus callosum, ⑤ caudate nucleus, ⑥ lentiform nucleus, ⑦ thalamus. ⊛ Branches of the anterior cerebral arteries.

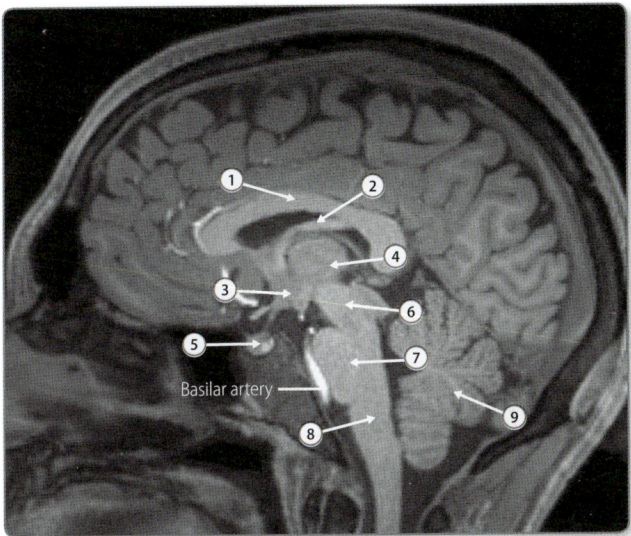

Figure 2.18 Mid-sagittal T1-weighted MRI scan, showing the medial surface of the brain. ① Corpus callosum, ② fornix, ③ hypothalamus, ④ thalamus, ⑤ pituitary gland, ⑥ midbrain, ⑦ pons, ⑧ medulla, ⑨ cerebellum.

The higher spatial resolution of MRI allows better visualisation of the cerebellar lobes and the folia. The appearance of cerebellar grey and white matter follows the same principles as described for the cerebrum.

2.6 The spinal cord

Whereas CT is preferred for visualising the spinal column (bone), MRI is preferred for the spinal cord and the nerve roots, because of its superior spatial resolution (**Figures 2.19** and **2.20**). The relation between the different MRI sequences and the appearance of different tissues follows the same principles as described for the brain (see **Table 2.2**). Generally, T1-weighted imaging is used to appreciate the anatomy of the spinal cord, and T2-weighted imaging to examine pathology.

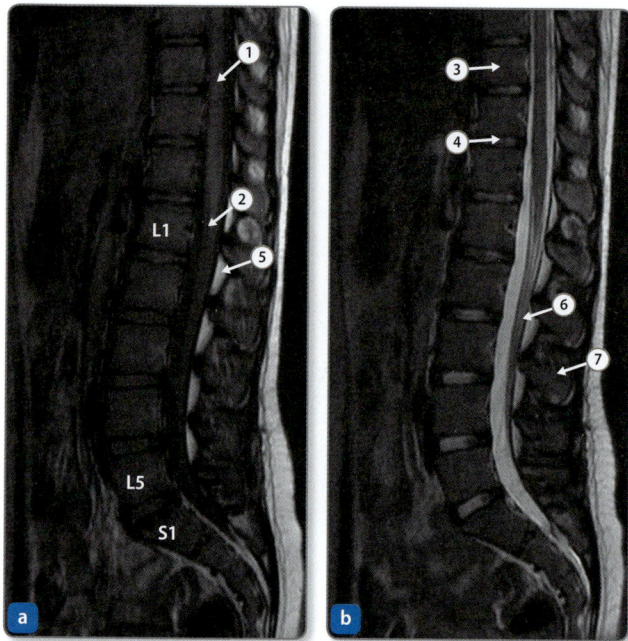

Figure 2.19 MRI scans of the lumbar sacral spine: (a) T1-weighted and (b) T2-weighted. ① Spinal cord, ② conus medullaris, ③ vertebral body, ④ intervertebral disc, ⑤ posterior epidural fat, ⑥ cauda equina (surrounded by cerebrospinal fluid in the lumbar cistern), ⑦ spinous processes.

2.7 The vasculature

On both CT and MRI, vessels appear circular when viewed through the lumen (examples shown in **Figure 2.17**), and as lines or curves when viewed from the side (examples shown in **Figure 2.18**).

CT

Large vessels are visible as hyperdense structures on CT. However, small vessels are difficult to discern, because of the limited spatial resolution offered by this imaging modality.

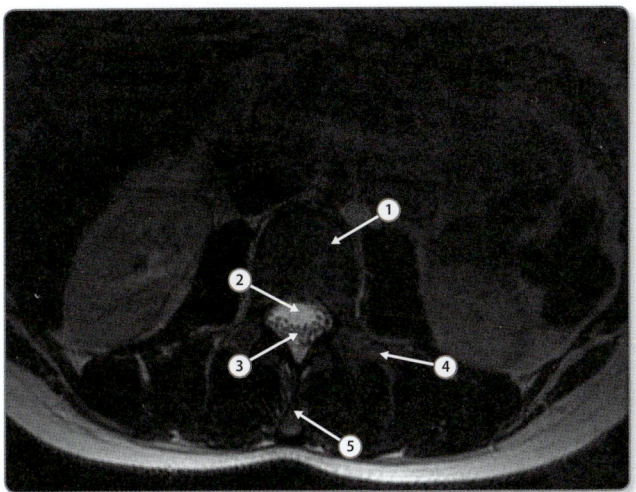

Figure 2.20 Axial T2-weighted MRI scan of a lumbar vertebra. ①Vertebral body, ②lumbar cistern, ③cauda equina, ④transverse process, ⑤spinous process.

Contrast media is used to improve visualisation of the vascular system. If images are acquired soon after the injection of contrast (in the 'arterial phase'), the arterial system is enhanced. The surrounding tissue can then be digitally removed to produce an image of the arterial system in isolation, i.e. a CT angiogram (**Figure 2.21**). If images are acquired later (in the 'venous phase'), the venous system is enhanced. Digital removal of the surrounding tissue produces an image of the venous system, i.e. the CT venogram.

MRI

The arterial system can be visualised by using magnetic resonance angiography, with or without gadolinium contrast

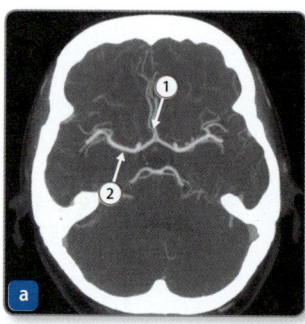

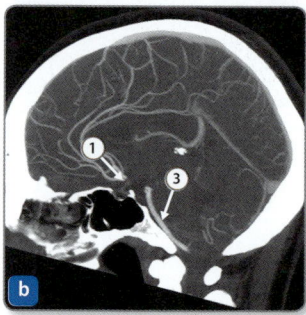

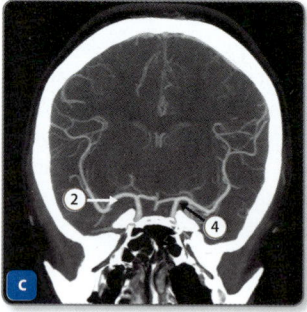

Figure 2.21 CT angiograms demonstrating cranial vasculature. (a) axial, (b) sagittal and (c) coronal sections. ① Anterior cerebral arteries, ② right middle cerebral artery, ③ basilar artery, ④ internal carotid artery.

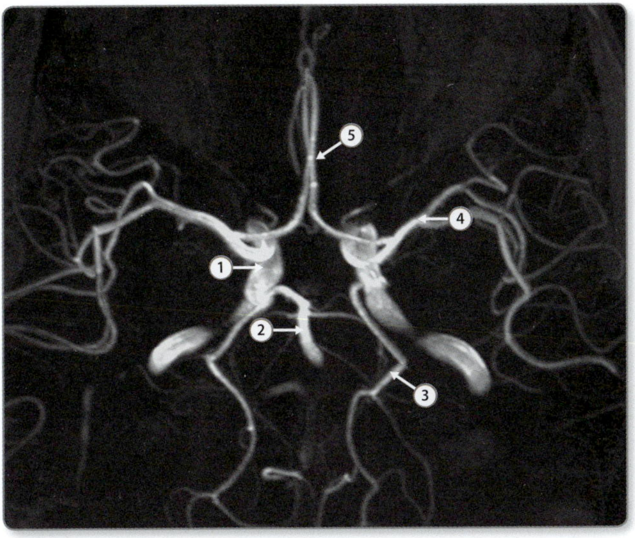

Figure 2.22 Magnetic resonance angiogram showing the circle of Willis.
① Internal carotid artery, ② basilar artery, ③ posterior cerebral artery,
④ middle cerebral artery, ⑤ anterior cerebral artery.

(**Figure 2.22**). In this technique, based on MRI, the signal of flowing blood is increased, and an image of the arterial system is produced by digital removal of surrounding tissues. Fast-flowing blood may appear as a hypointense flow void.

In magnetic resonance venography, image acquisition is delayed until the venous phase. The resulting image shows the venous system.

Digital subtraction angiography

Digital subtraction angiography is a fluoroscopy technique that uses contrast and serial ('real-time') plain radiographs to image the flow of blood through the vessels of the brain. Initially the arterial system will be seen and then the venous system

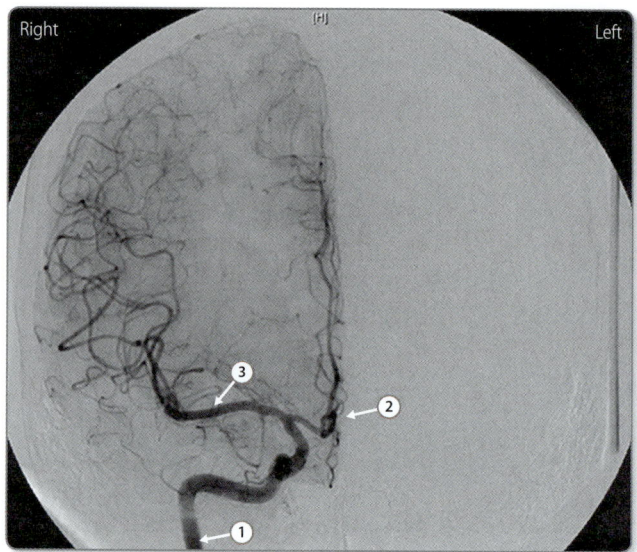

Figure 2.23 Anteroposterior digital subtraction angiogram showing the right internal carotid artery and its branches. ① Internal carotid artery, ② anterior cerebral artery, ③ middle cerebral artery.

afterwards. Digital subtraction angiography can be used to diagnose vascular malformations or to guide procedures that treat vascular malformations (such as coiling of an aneurysm).

Angiography is carried out by inserting a catheter into the arterial system, usually from a common femoral puncture, manipulating the catheter into the artery of choice (the common or internal carotid artery or the vertebral artery), then injecting iodinated contrast and obtaining digital radiographic images of its vascular distribution. Images acquired in the arterial or venous phase show the arterial and venous distribution, respectively. Digital subtraction of surrounding tissues is then used to make the vasculature more conspicuous (**Figures 2.23** and **2.24**).

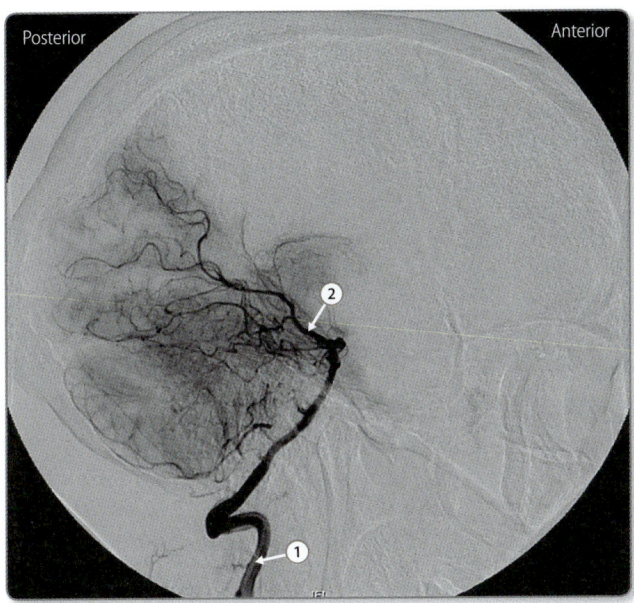

Figure 2.24 Lateral digital subtraction angiogram showing the right vertebral artery and its branches. ① Vertebral artery, ② posterior cerebral artery.

2.8 Cerebrospinal fluid

CT

Compartments containing cerebrospinal fluid appear hypodense. These include the ventricles (**Figure 2.25**), the sub-arachnoid space (including the cisterns, **Figure 2.26**) and the sulci. Within the lateral ventricles, the choroid plexus, where cerebrospinal fluid is produced, may appear hyperdense on CT as a consequence of calcification.

Clinical insight

The ventricular system is morphologically variable within the normal population. The ability to recognise abnormalities requires experience of viewing many normal images in addition to an understanding of the anatomy.

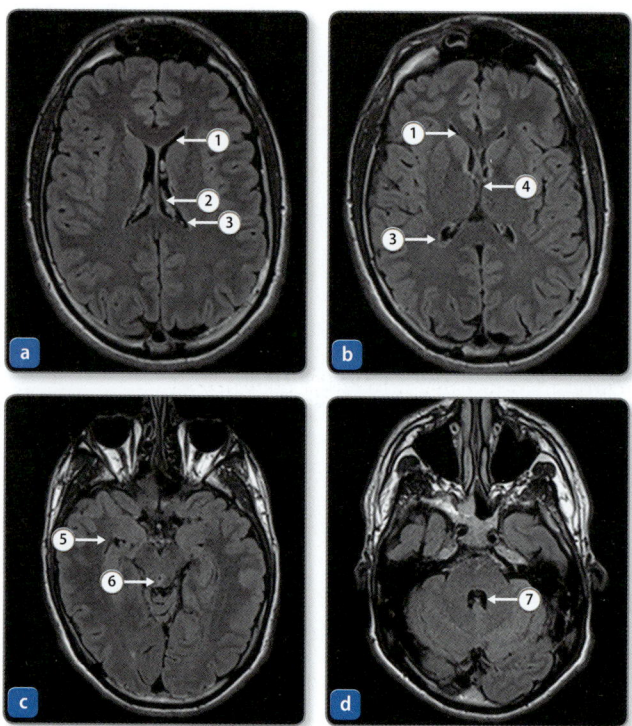

Figure 2.25 T2–FLAIR MRI scans showing the ventricular system (in order of superior to inferior). ① Frontal horn of the lateral ventricle, ② choroid plexus of the lateral ventricle, ③ occipital horn of the lateral ventricle, ④ interventricular foramen (of Munro) ⑤ temporal horn of the lateral ventricle, ⑥ cerebral aqueduct (of Sylvius), ⑦ fourth ventricle.

MRI

Cerebrospinal fluid appears hypointense on T1-weighted MRI, and hyperintense on T2-weighted MRI. It appears hypointense on T2–FLAIR (see **Figure 2.25**). T2–FLAIR is useful when assessing for pathology at the boundary of the ventricles and the parenchyma.

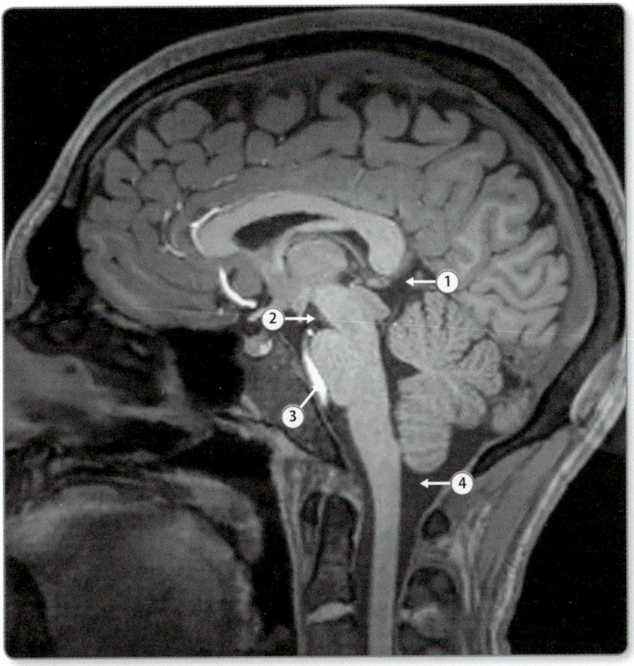

Figure 2.26 Mid-sagittal T1-weighted MRI scan showing the basal cisterns. (1) Quadrigeminal cistern, (2) interpeduncular cistern, (3) pontine cistern, (4) cisterna magna.

Interpreting abnormal images

3.1 Fractures

Fractures of the skull and spine are covered in Chapters 4 and 9, respectively.

3.2 Intracranial haemorrhage

Haemorrhage is the extravasation of blood from the breached vascular system. A haematoma is an internal accumulation of blood in a relatively or completely closed space, as a consequence of haemorrhage.

Blood can accumulate in various compartments within the cranium (**Figure 3.1**), and intracranial haemorrhages are described in terms of their location. As with other neurological pathologies, it is important to state whether the haemorrhage appears extra-axial or intra-axial, because this helps to narrow down the differential diagnosis.

CT

A clot formed due to acute haemorrhage typically appears hyperdense on CT in comparison with surrounding parenchyma, but as the blood degrades it becomes less bright and thus iso- and then hypo-dense on CT. This is how we may predict the age of a haemorrhage, classifying it radiologically as acute, subacute, chronic or acute-on-chronic (see Figures 4.6–4.10). However, a caveat is that active bleeding (rather than clotted blood) will appear as an intermediate or low density area and could be misidentified.

> **Clinical insight**
>
> An intra-axial feature is one that is within the parenchyma of the brain. An extra-axial feature is one that is outside the parenchyma. For example, an intraparenchymal brain haemorrhage is an intra-axial lesion, whereas a subdural haematoma is an extra-axial lesion.

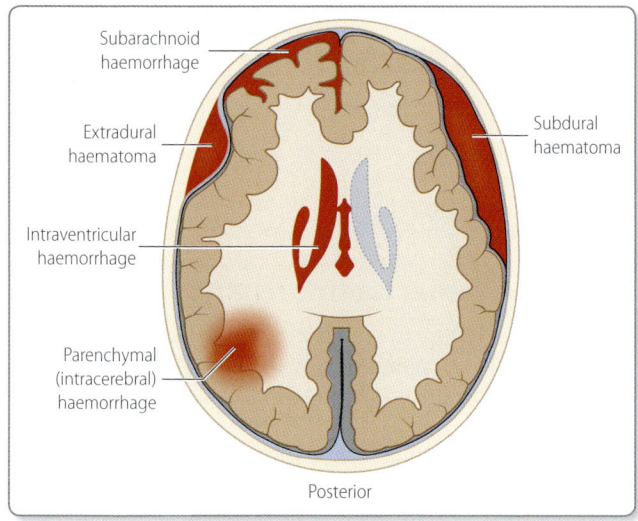

Figure 3.1 Types of intracranial haemorrhage.

MRI

As on CT, the appearance of blood on MRI changes over time (**Figure 3.2**). Its imaging characteristics also differ depending on the MRI sequence used. Specialist MRI sequences that are useful for detecting blood include T2-weighted gradient echo and susceptibility-weighted imaging.

3.3 Ischaemia

Ischaemia is a disturbance of cellular function resulting from inadequate blood supply. Prolonged ischaemia may produce an infarct, i.e. an area of dead tissue. The radiological features of ischaemia and infarction are described in Chapter 5.

3.4 Cerebral oedema

Cerebral oedema is caused by increased fluid within the cerebral parenchyma. It is not a diagnosis but rather the consequence

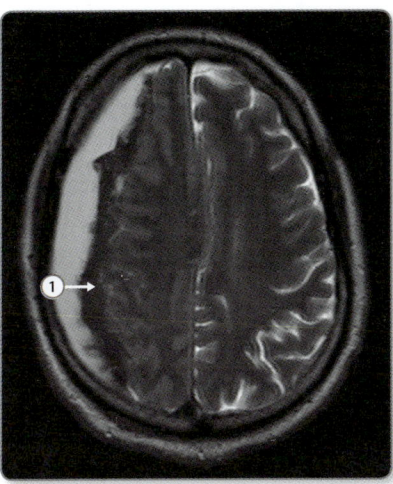

Figure 3.2 Axial T2-weighted MRI scan showing a right acute-on-chronic subdural haematoma. ① Low signal intensity in the deep margin probably indicates recent haemorrhage.

of underlying pathology. The characteristic features of the different types of cerebral oedema are shown in **Figure 3.3** and summarised in **Table 3.1**.

3.5 Hydrocephalus

Hydrocephalus is an abnormal increase in the volume of cerebrospinal fluid contained within the ventricular system. As hydrocephalus progresses, the ventricular system becomes dilatated (termed ventriculomegaly; **Figure 3.4**), and intracranial pressure increases. Excessive intracranial pressure forces cerebrospinal fluid into the periventricular white matter (transependymal flow) to produce transependymal oedema (see **Table 3.1**).

Hydrocephalus is generally divided into communicating and non-communicating (or obstructive) hydrocephalus. In this context, 'communicating' means that the cerebrospinal fluid can continue to flow through the ventricles, which remain patent.

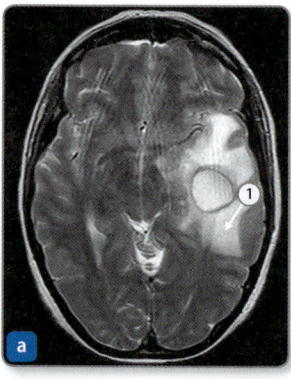

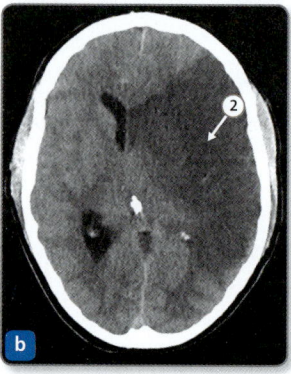

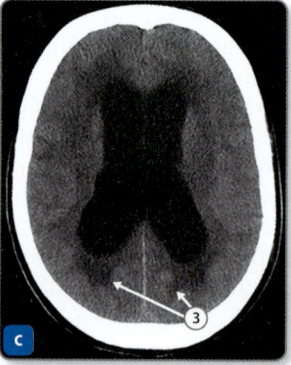

Figure 3.3 Features of different types of cerebral oedema. (a) Axial T2-weighted MRI scan showing vasogenic oedema ① in a cerebral abscess. (b) Axial CT scan showing cytotoxic oedema ② in malignant middle cerebral artery syndrome. (c) Axial CT scan showing transependymal oedema ③ in hydrocephalus.

Characteristic	Vasogenic oedema	Cytotoxic oedema	Transependymal oedema
Mechanism	Disruption of blood–brain barrier Fluid collects in extracellular space	Disruption of membrane's ability to balance fluid between intra- and extracellular spaces Fluid collects in intracellular space	Increased pressure in ventricular system forces fluid across ependymal lining and into surrounding brain parenchyma
CT appearance	Hypodensity Increased grey and white matter differentiation	Hypodensity Loss of grey and white matter differentiation	Hypodensity adjacent to lateral ventricles
MRI appearance	T2-weighted and T2–FLAIR: high signal	T1- or T2-weighted: no change DWI: high signal ADC: low signal	T2-weighted and T2–FLAIR: high signal surrounding lateral ventricles
Examples of underlying pathology	Brain tumours Cerebral infections (including abscesses) Parenchymal brain haemorrhage	Ischaemic stroke Traumatic brain injury	Hydrocephalus
ADC, apparent diffusion coefficient; DWI, diffusion-weighed imaging.			

Table 3.1 Comparison of types of oedema

Communicating hydrocephalus

Communicating hydrocephalus is caused by an imbalance between the production and absorption of cerebrospinal fluid. The most common causes are meningitis and subarachnoid haemorrhage.

Normal pressure hydrocephalus

Normal pressure hydrocephalus is a poorly understood type of communicating hydrocephalus. As the name implies, there

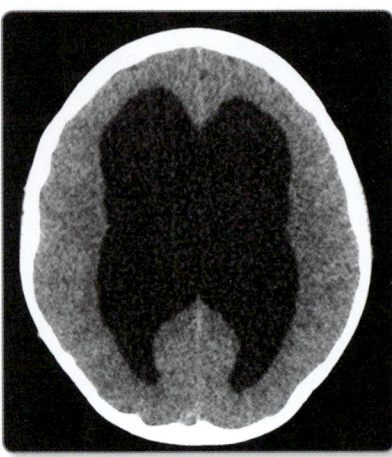

Figure 3.4 Axial CT scan from a patient with hydrocephalus. The lateral ventricles are grossly enlarged.

is an increased volume of cerebrospinal fluid and consequent ventriculomegaly; however, there is no sustained increase in intracranial pressure.

Non-communicating hydrocephalus

Non-communicating hydrocephalus occurs when cerebrospinal fluid outflow is obstructed. It is caused by any space-occupying lesion or stenosis that blocks the passage of cerebrospinal fluid through the ventricular system. Since cerebrospinal fluid flows through the ventricular system from superior to inferior, ventriculomegaly occurs superior to the point of obstruction (**Figure 3.5**).

3.6 Increased intracranial pressure

In adults, the intracranial cavity has a fixed volume. Therefore, the presence of a space-occupying lesion (e.g. a haematoma or tumour) may lead to increased intracranial pressure and displacement of intracranial contents.

Features of increased intracranial pressure on neuroimaging are (**Figure 3.6**):

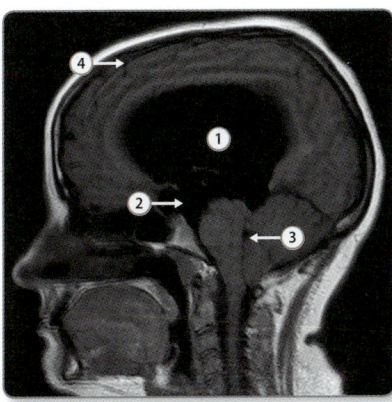

Figure 3.5 Sagittal T1-weighted MRI scan from a patient with congenital aqueduct stenosis. (1) Dilatated lateral ventricle, (2) dilatated third ventricle, (3) normal fourth ventricle, (4) motion artefact.

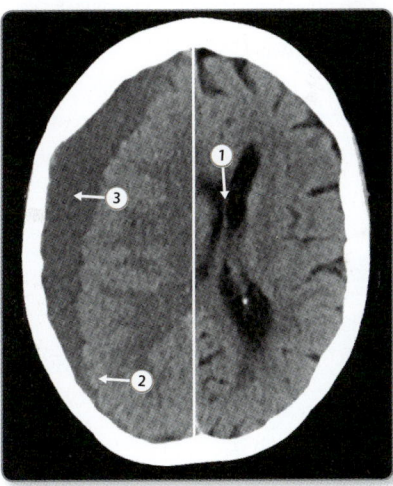

Figure 3.6 Axial CT scan showing a subdural haematoma causing mass effect and increased intracranial pressure. (1) Midline shift, (2) effacement of the sulci, (3) right chronic subdural haematoma. The white line shows the midline of the brain.

- Effacement of the sulci (the cerebrospinal fluid space between the sulci is no longer seen)
- Compression of the ventricles
- Midline shift
- Effacement of the basal cisterns
- Herniation

Herniation occurs when part of the brain is forced from its normal location into a different anatomical space (**Figure 3.7**). Subfalcine herniation occurs when the cingulate gyrus is

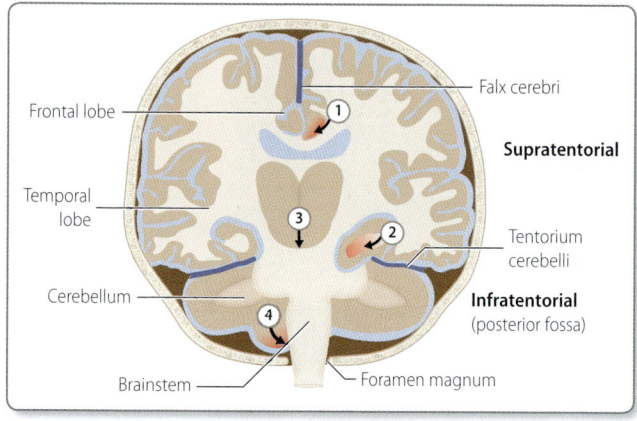

Figure 3.7 Sites of brain herniation. ① Subfalcine herniation, ② transtentorial (uncal) herniation, ③ central herniation, ④ tonsillar herniation (true coning).

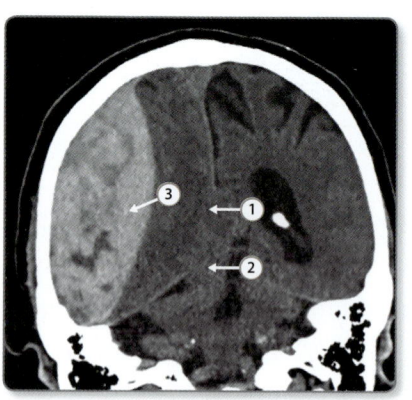

Figure 3.8 Coronal CT scan showing subfalcine herniation ① and transtentorial herniation ② caused by a haematoma ③.

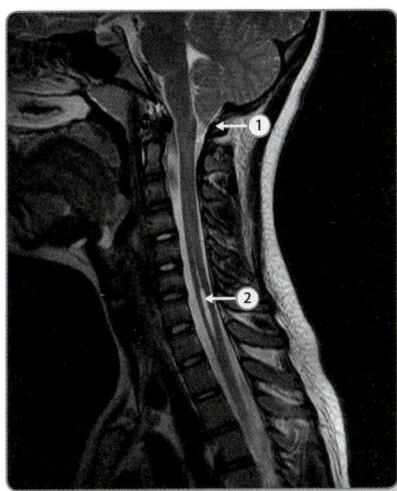

Figure 3.9 Sagittal T2-weighted MRI scan of the posterior fossa and cervical spine, showing a type 1 Chiari malformation. ① Herniation of the cerebellar tonsils through the foramen magnum, ② syrinx.

displaced under the falx cerebri (**Figure 3.8**). Uncal herniation, also known as descending transtentorial herniation, occurs when the uncus of the temporal lobe is displaced over the edge of the tentorium cerebelli (**Figure 3.8**).

Tonsillar herniation is the process by which the cerebellar tonsils are forced to descend through the foramen magnum. It is a late and grave feature of increased intracranial pressure. A non-life-threatening example of chronic tonsillar herniation is a type 1 Chiari malformation (**Figure 3.9**).

3.7 Abnormal presence of air

In neuroimaging, air may be detected in the extracranial soft tissue (subcutaneous emphysema) or within the cranium (pneumocephalus). Pneumocephalus develops in response to a breach of the skull, common causes of which include fracture, infection or surgery (**Figure 3.10**). Pneumocephalus may either be extra- or intra-axial.

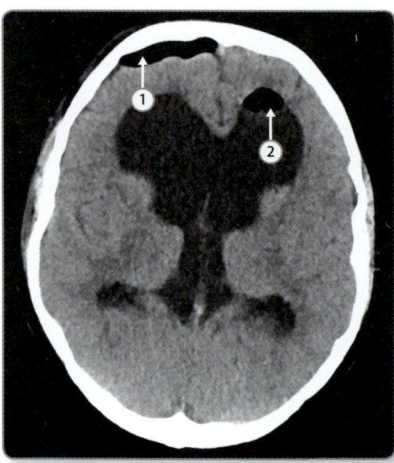

Figure 3.10 Axial CT scan showing pneumocephalus at the frontal pole ① and within the left lateral ventricle ②.

3.8 Features of ageing

In images of the elderly brain there are several features that appear abnormal but are considered features of normal ageing rather than signs of disease. They are variable within the population, and are not always present.

Cortical atrophy

This is a very common finding in elderly patients, and reflects decreases in the size and number of brain cells. It is evident on CT and MRI as prominent sulci (**Figure 3.11**).

In addition to normal ageing, cortical atrophy can develop secondary to pathological causes, including degenerative neurological conditions such as Alzheimer's disease.

Ventriculomegaly

Ventriculomegaly can develop because of generalised brain atrophy. There is apparent ventriculomegaly but no change in intraventricular pressure.

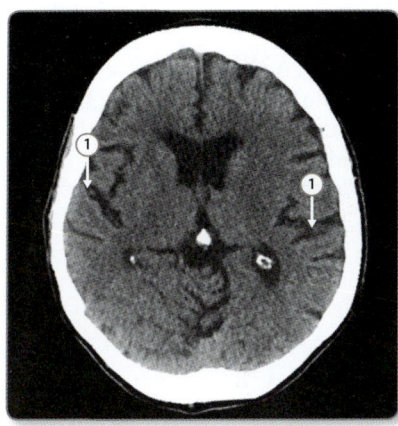

Figure 3.11 Axial CT scan from a patient with dementia. There is generalised atrophy, resulting in prominent sulci ①.

Small vessel disease

Small vessel disease is a multifactorial cerebrovascular disorder. On neuroimaging, it is indicated by evidence of:

- lacunar infarcts
- microbleeds
- white matter lesions
- perivascular Virchow–Robin spaces (visible, fluid-filled spaces between small arteries and the brain) and
- brain atrophy

These pathological changes are most apparent on MRI.

3.9 Incidental findings

Incidental findings are features found on imaging that are of potential clinical importance but discovered unintentionally. They are relatively common, occurring in about 1 in 40 asymptomatic people. However, active intervention is required in only a small minority of cases.

An example of an incidental finding is shown in Figure 4.6. A meningioma was discovered as an incidental finding on CT after a traumatic brain injury.

3.10 Artefact

It is common to find features on neuroimaging that are attributable to radiographic errors or the limitations of the technology, and therefore do not reflect the true structure of the brain or spinal cord. These features are called artefacts.

There are many types of artefact. Some of the most common are caused by:

- foreign bodies

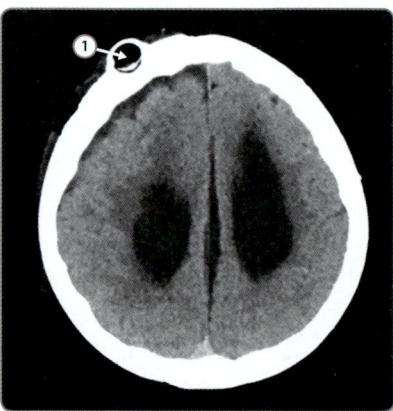

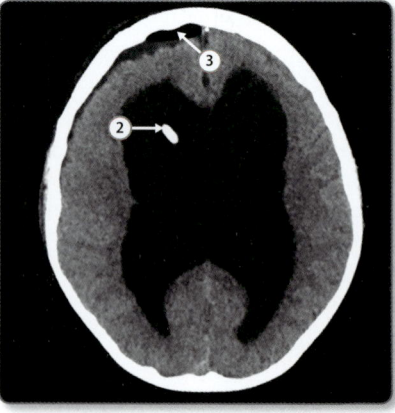

Figure 3.12 Axial CT scan showing a foreign body: an Ommaya reservoir ① and its ventricular catheter ②. ③ Pneumocephalus.

- metal
- patient movement and
- scattering of X-ray beams

Foreign bodies

Foreign bodies that may appear on neuroimaging include:

- dentures

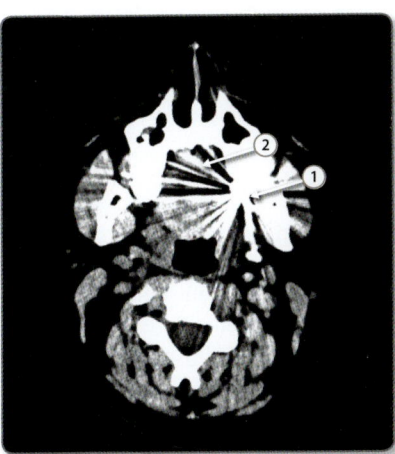

Figure 3.13 Axial CT scan at the level of the teeth, showing a metal foreign body ① and starburst artefact ②.

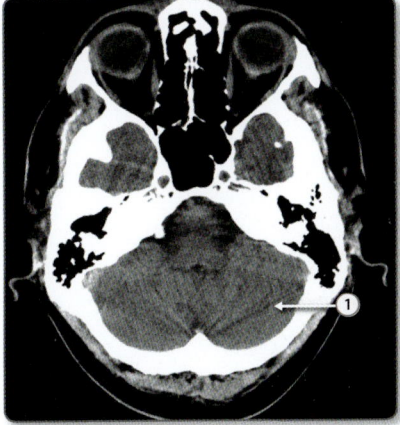

Figure 3.14 Axial CT scan of the brainstem and cerebellum, showing beam hardening artefact ① between dense skull.

- aneurysm clips and
- devices for diverting cerebrospinal fluid (**Figure 3.12**)

Starburst

Metal foreign bodies cause starburst artefact, named after its distinctive appearance on CT. Bright and dark streaks radiate from the location of the metal object (**Figure 3.13**).

Motion

Motion artefact is the distortion of a radiological image caused by movement of the patient (**Figure 3.5**). It is more of a problem in MRI than in CT, because image acquisition takes longer in MRI. However, it can hinder the interpretation of images obtained with either modality.

Beam hardening

The CT artefact of beam hardening (or scattering) is the consequence of miscalculation of the range of Hounsfield units used when obtaining images of tissue between dense structures. Bright or dark lines may appear between different parts of the skull, particularly around the skull base (**Figure 3.14**).

Trauma

Most head injuries sustained are minor and their effects short lasting, but in some the injury is severe enough to damage the brain and disrupt its normal function; this is known as traumatic brain injury. It can have devastating lifelong effects, and is associated with a high mortality rate. Traumatic brain injury is common both in the UK (an incidence of around 500 in 100,000 people per year) and on a global scale.

In the UK and other high-income countries, traumatic brain injury has a bimodal age distribution. The groups most likely to sustain a brain injury are young men (through risk-taking behaviour or violence) and elderly people (from falls).

Traumatic brain injury is characterised clinically according to the patient's Glasgow Coma Scale (GCS) score.

- Minor (GCS score 13–15)
- Moderate (GCS score 9–12)
- Severe (GCS score 3–8)

The pathophysiology of traumatic brain injury is divided into:

- **Primary**: if the injury was sustained at the time of trauma
- **Secondary**: if the injury evolved over time as a consequence of progression of a cascade of maladaptive physiological responses (including oedema, inflammation)

Primary prevention measures, such as speed limits for road traffic, are used to reduce the incidence of primary traumatic brain injury. The prevention of secondary brain injury relies on the input of pre-hospital medicine, emergency department trauma care, neurosurgeons and intensive care.

4.1 Clinical scenario

Loss of consciousness after an assault

Presentation

A 22-year-old man is brought to the emergency department after being assaulted outside a nightclub. His friend is present and reports that he was badly beaten and then 'knocked out' by a punch to the side of the head but had regained consciousness initially. The paramedics report that his GCS score has been decreasing during transfer to the emergency department. On examination, GCS score is E1 V2 M4, and he has a right dilated pupil that is not reactive to light.

Initial interpretation

In this context, a fixed dilated pupil indicates a third nerve palsy caused by life-threatening traumatic brain injury and brain herniation. After the patient has been resuscitated using the ABCDE approach, CT of the head is immediately required.

Imaging findings

The most striking abnormality on the CT scan is a large, space-occupying, extra-axial right-sided collection (**Figure 4.1**). There are two different components. The first is a superficial, biconvex, hyper- or mixed-density collection that is restricted by suture lines. The second is a deeper, crescentic (crescent moon-shaped), hyperdense collection that does not appear to be restricted by suture lines. There is evidence of mass effect, with right-to-left

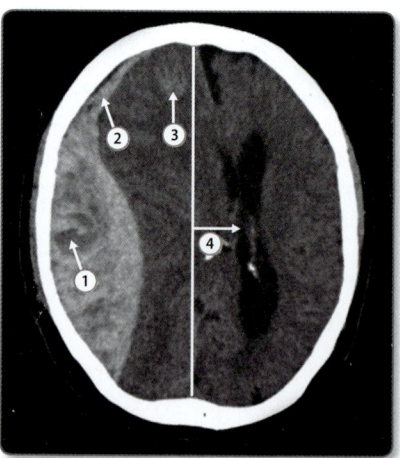

Figure 4.1 Axial CT scan showing traumatic brain injury. ① Extradural haematoma, ② acute subdural haematoma, ③ frontal lobe contusion, ④ midline shift.

midline shift. An intra-axial hyperdense lesion is visible in the right frontal lobe.

Diagnosis

The imaging findings confirm that this patient has sustained a severe traumatic brain injury. This includes a right extradural haematoma, right acute subdural haematoma and right frontal contusion.

> ### Clinical insight
>
> This clinical scenario describes an example of trauma generating multiple pathologies. In traumatic brain injury, it is essential to carefully examine the results of imaging studies for additional pathology. This includes using the CT bone window to search for skull fractures.

Management

Urgent craniotomy and decompression are required, alongside neurointensive care, to reduce the intracranial pressure and remove the haematoma.

4.2 Approach to the trauma patient

Assessment

In any trauma case, the priority is resuscitation of the patient. This begins with the airway, breathing, circulation, disability and exposure (ABCDE) approach, which prioritises assessment and intervention in the acute management of a trauma patient. The cervical spine should be secured immediately.

Assessment of disability requires a focused review of the patient's conscious level (using the GCS; **Table 4.1**), examination of the pupils, and if possible, examination for focal neurological signs. If the GCS score is 8 or less, assistance from a senior doctor with expertise in maintaining an airway is required, as well as immediate discussion with the on-call neurosurgeon.

Role of neuroimaging

Once the patient is clinically stable, the first radiological investigation is an urgent non-contrast CT scan of the head.

Plain radiography Skull radiographs are no longer acquired for head injury; they have been superseded by CT. Cervical spine injuries are covered in section 9.2.

Score	Eye response	Verbal response	Motor response
6	–	–	Follows commands
5	–	Oriented	Localising
4	Spontaneous	Confused	Normal flexion
3	To sound	Words	Abnormal flexion
2	To pressure	Sounds	Extension
1	None	None	None

Table 4.1 Glasgow Coma Scale for adults. The patient is given a score for each category: eyes, voice and motor. 15 is the maximum score and 3 is the minimum score

CT This is the imaging modality of choice in traumatic brain injury; image acquisition is more rapid than with MRI. Also, MRI is inappropriate as a first-line investigation in trauma, because it cannot be assured that the patient is free from MRI-incompatible implants or ferromagnetic material introduced into the body in a penetrating injury.

Indications for an immediate CT head scan after head injury include:
- GCS score less than 13 on initial assessment
- GCS score less than 15, 2 hours after admission to the emergency department
- Suspected open or depressed skull fracture
- Any sign of basal skull fracture
- Post-traumatic seizure
- Focal neurological deficit
- More than one episode of vomiting since the head injury

Indications for a CT head scan within 8 hours of head injury include:
- Age over 65 years
- A coagulation disorder, or use of warfarin
- Dangerous mechanism of injury (e.g. a fall down more than five stairs, or more than 1 metre)
- More than 30 minutes of retrograde amnesia of preinjury events

Differential diagnoses

Table 4.2 lists the common presentations in traumatic brain injury and other diagnoses to consider.

Presentation	Differential diagnoses	Initial imaging required
Any patient presenting after traumatic head injury	Soft tissue injury Skull fracture Extradural haematoma Subdural haematoma Subarachnoid haemorrhage Parenchymal brain haemorrhage haemorrhage or contusions Diffuse axonal injury	CT head CT cervical spine
Patient found in coma	Traumatic brain injury (as above) Infection (e.g. meningitis) Vascular disease (e.g. brainstem stroke) Endocrine disease (e.g. hypoglycaemia) Drug overdose (of prescription or non-prescription drugs) Metabolic encephalopathy (alcohol poisoning) Seizures	CT head Also CT cervical spine (if trauma suspected)
Patient with cerebrospinal fluid rhinorrhoea or haemotympanum	Basal skull fracture	CT head
Elderly patient with confusion progressing over weeks	Chronic subdural haematoma Delirium (e.g. caused by UTI) Dementia Cerebral tumour Normal pressure hydrocephalus	CT head
Patient with a head injury, initial unconsciousness, a lucid interval, then finally persistent unconsciousness	Extradural haematoma (classic presentation) Other traumatic brain injuries must be excluded	CT head CT cervical spine

Table 4.2 Traumatic brain injury: differential diagnoses according to presentation. UTI, urinary tract infection

4.3 Skull fracture

Skull fractures are described in terms of location, pattern and skin integrity.

- Fractures can occur at the skull vault or at the skull base (basal fracture)
- The pattern of fracture is linear (single fracture line) or comminuted (with several fracture lines)
- Fractures may be depressed (bone is displaced towards the brain)
- Fractures are either open (skin integrity is compromised) or closed (skin integrity is not compromised)

Key facts

- With a suspected skull fracture, clinical examination of the skull should be attempted with caution, to avoid causing further injury
- Clinical features suggesting a basal skull fracture of the anterior cranial fossa include cerebrospinal fluid rhinorrhoea, bilateral periorbital ecchymoses (bruising, raccoon or panda eyes) and subconjunctival haemorrhage
- Clinical features suggesting a fracture of the middle cranial fossa include blood in the tympanic cavity of the ear (haemotympanum), cerebrospinal fluid otorrhoea and ecchymoses over the mastoid (Battle's sign)
- Complications of skull fracture include pneumocephalus (air within the cranial cavity), meningitis and sepsis. Basal skull fractures are associated with neurological deficits and vascular injuries. Fractures through the temporal bone and inner ear may lead to sensorineuronal deafness

Imaging findings

Indications for an imaging study for a suspected skull fracture include:

- Clinical suspicion of an open or depressed skull fracture
- Signs of a basal skull fracture

CT This is the preferred imaging modality for identifying skull fractures. When a bone window is used, skull fractures appear as hypodense lines (**Figure 4.2**). In comminuted fractures, several fracture lines and bone fragments are visible (**Figure 4.3**). Depressed fractures appear as sections of bone that are displaced deep to the adjacent skull (**Figure 4.4**).

A thorough search for any intracranial haemorrhage is essential because fractures are frequently associated with extradural, subdural or subarachnoid haemorrhages. Soft tissue injury or haematoma may also be present.

Skull base fractures are subtle. The mastoid air cells require thorough evaluation. In adults, the mastoid air cells are normally completely aerated; opacification in the context of trauma raises the suspicion of fracture.

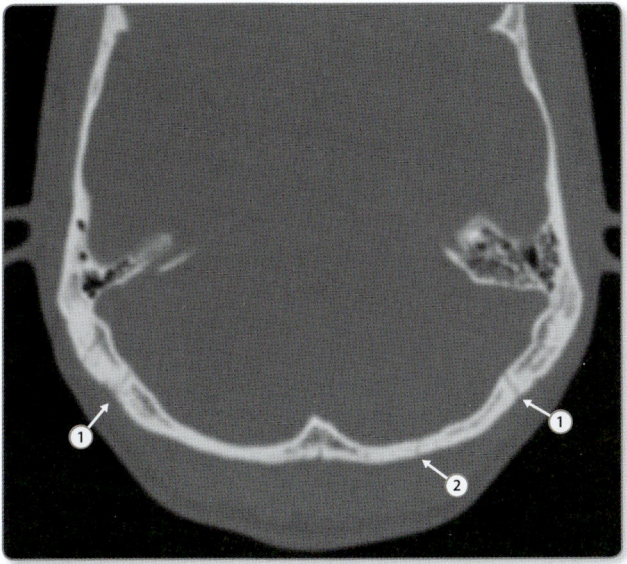

Figure 4.2 Axial CT scan (bone window) showing a skull fracture. ① Right and left lambdoid suture lines, ② fracture line on the left side of the occipital bone.

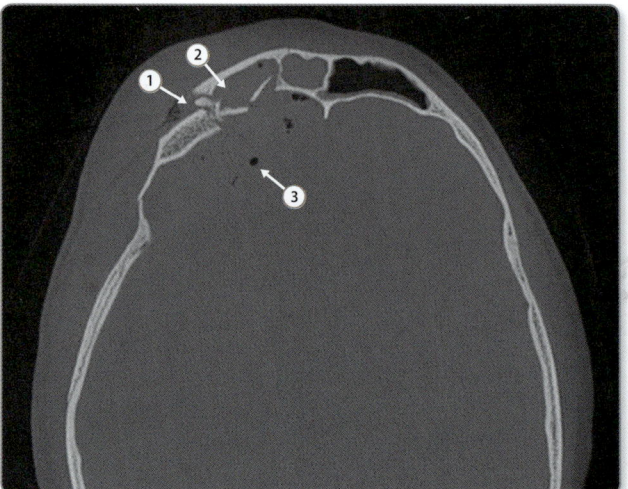

Figure 4.3 Axial CT scan (bone window) showing a comminuted fracture.
① Fracture of the frontal bone, with involvement of the frontal sinus,
② effusion or haemorrhage within the frontal sinus, ③ pneumocephalus.

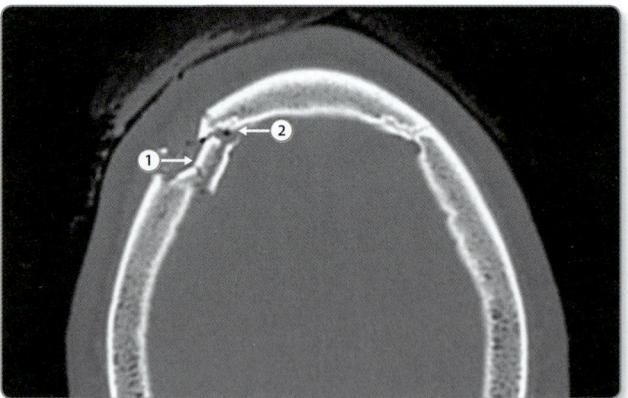

Figure 4.4 Axial CT scan (bone window) showing a depressed skull fracture.
① Depressed fracture, ② pneumocephalus.

Foreign bodies should be searched for, if appropriate given the mechanism of injury. Metallic objects may appear as a starburst artefact (see section 3.10). Scalp haematoma superficial to the fracture appears as a crescentic mass of intermediate density.

Pneumocephalus is identified by the presence of small spherical hypodensities within the cranium. These tend to be superficial rather than deep (see **Figure 4.4**), and represent air bubbles.

Management

The management of skull fractures requires discussion with the neurosurgical team, because surgical intervention is occasionally required. Neurosurgical intervention may be indicated for an open skull fracture, significant depressed fracture and fracture associated with neurological deficit or cerebrospinal fluid leak.

4.4 Extradural haematoma

An extradural (or epidural) haematoma is an accumulation of blood superficial to the dura mater and deep to the skull. It is extra-axial, because it lies outside the brain parenchyma.

Key facts

- Typical mechanisms of injury producing extradural haematoma include road traffic accidents, assault and falls
- Extradural haematoma is typically caused by fractures of the squamous part of the temporal bone, resulting in rupture of the middle meningeal artery
- Extradural haematomas may also arise from bleeding of the venous sinuses
- The classic history for an extradural haematoma is loss of consciousness at the time of injury, restoration of

consciousness for a short period of lucency, and then progression to unconsciousness as the haematoma expands
- Expansion of the haematoma causes increased intracranial pressure and mass effect (see section 3.6)

Imaging findings

CT An extradural haematoma appears as an extra-axial biconvex lesion, typically in the temporoparietal zone (see **Figure 4.1**), although variations occur (**Figure 4.5**). The lesion appears hyperdense, because of the acute accumulation of clotted blood. The dura mater is adherent to the periosteum at the sutures, so an extradural haematoma seldom crosses these lines.

Extradural haematomas are associated with skull fractures. Therefore, inspection of skull integrity on CT with bone window is essential.

Management

As with any case of head injury, the priority is resuscitation, for which a systematic ABCDE approach is used. Extradural haematoma should always be discussed with an on-call neurosurgeon.

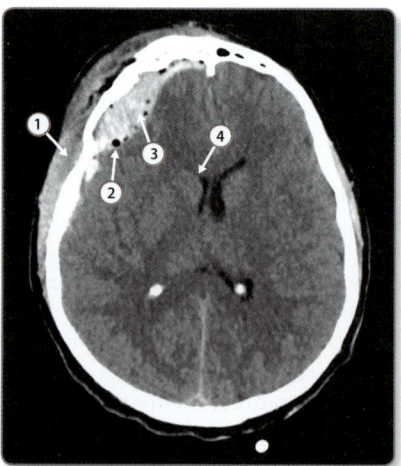

Figure 4.5 Axial CT showing an extradural haematoma. ① Soft tissue haematoma, ② pneumocephalus, ③ right frontal convexity extradural haematoma underlying a frontal bone fracture (corresponding with the fracture in Figure 4.3), ④ effacement of the right frontal horn of the lateral ventricle.

Indications for surgical management are based on the size of the haematoma and the neurological status of the patient. If surgery is required, a craniotomy is carried out and the haematoma evacuated. Temporalising preoperative measures, such as osmotic therapy (hypertonic saline or mannitol), may be recommended by the neurosurgeon.

4.5 Subdural haematoma

A subdural haematoma is a collection of blood that accumulates between the dura mater and the subarachnoid mater.

Key facts
- Subdural haematoma is a heterogeneous condition, with varying causative mechanisms, pathophysiology and sequelae
- It is classified clinically according to the time between head injury and presentation: acute (less than 4 days), subacute (4–21 days) and chronic (more than 21 days)
- It is classified radiologically according to imaging features: acute, subacute, chronic, or acute on chronic
- Acute subdural haematoma is most commonly caused by trauma. There is a spectrum of severity; a small, non-expanding acute subdural haematoma may be asymptomatic, whereas a large or expanding acute subdural haematoma may cause significant mass effect and increased intracranial pressure. Acute subdural haematoma may be accompanied by severe parenchymal injury
- Chronic subdural haematoma typically occurs because of tearing of the bridging veins that empty cortical blood into the venous sinuses; the resulting haematoma expands slowly, so presentation is late. Elderly patients are more susceptible, because the bridging veins are left vulnerable by age-related cortical atrophy. As well as old age, risk factors include use of anticoagulant medications, alcoholism and low intracranial pressure (e.g. from excessive drainage from ventriculoperitoneal shunting)

Imaging findings

Urgent imaging is required to confirm the diagnosis and assess the need for neurosurgical intervention.

CT Subdural haematomas are extra-axial, crescentic and not limited by suture lines.

- Acute subdural haematoma is apparent as a hyperdense lesion representing the collection of fresh blood (**Figure 4.6**)
- Chronic subdural haematoma appears hypodense, because the blood has had time to degrade (**Figure 4.7**). Chronic subdural haematoma may feature loculation and septation, with separated compartments of blood (**Figure 4.8**)
- In acute-on-chronic subdural haematoma, both acute and aged blood collections are visible. The collections of new and old blood may appear as a layered phenomenon, owing to the supine positioning of the patient in the CT scanner (**Figure 4.9**)

A subdural haematoma is termed isodense if it and the surrounding parenchyma are of equal density (**Figure 4.10**). These cases are less obvious and may be missed without careful inspection.

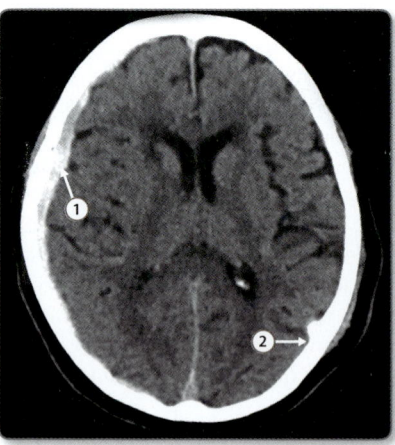

Figure 4.6 Axial CT scan showing a right acute subdural haematoma ①. ② Incidental left calcified lesion (most likely a calcified meningioma).

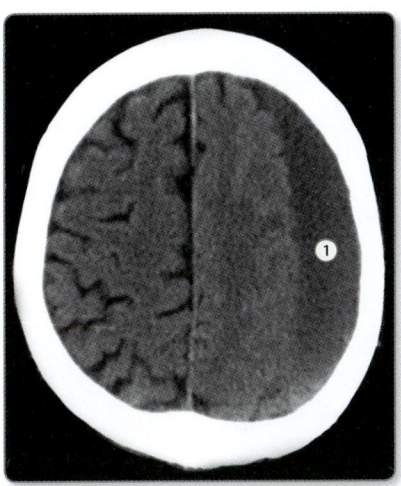

Figure 4.7 Axial CT scan showing a left chronic subdural haematoma ①. The haematoma appears hypodense.

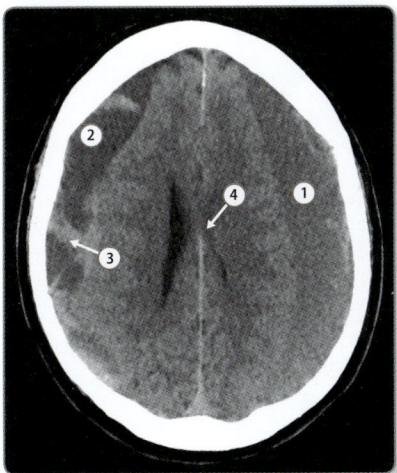

Figure 4.8 Axial CT scan of the head, showing bilateral chronic subdural haematoma. ① Left chronic subdural haematoma, ② right chronic subdural haematoma, ③ membranes, ④ mass effect causing compression of the ventricles.

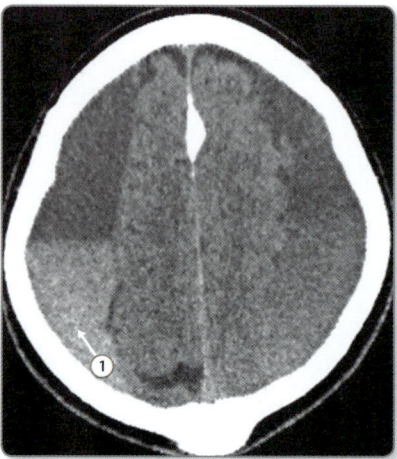

Figure 4.9 CT scan of bilateral subacute subdural haemorrhages. The right subdural haemorrhage demonstrates layering of blood ①.

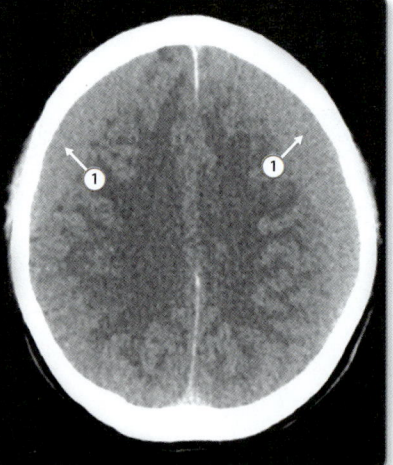

Figure 4.10 Axial CT scan showing bilateral isodense subdural haematomas ①.

Feature	Extradural haematoma	Subdural haematoma	
		Acute	Chronic
Morphology	Biconvex/lentiform	Crescentic	Crescentic
Density	Hyperdense	Hyperdense	Hypodense
Relation to suture lines	Does not cross	Crosses	Crosses
Relation to venous sinuses	Crosses	Does not cross	Does not cross

Table 4.3 Extradural and subdural haematoma: radiological differentiating features

In all types of subdural haematoma, mass effect may occur (see section 3.6). Elderly patients tend to accommodate far greater volumes of subdural haematoma, because age-related brain atrophy leaves more space for expansion.

The characteristic differences between the appearances of extradural and subdural haematoma are shown in **Table 4.3**.

Management

Not all subdural haematomas require surgery. The decision to operate is based on the clinical severity, the patient's comorbidities and the experienced opinion of the neurosurgeon. Surgical treatment consists of either burr hole drainage or craniotomy.

4.6 Cerebral contusion

Cerebral contusions are a form of intraparenchymal brain haemorrhage. They are injuries in which there is localised leakage of blood into the brain parenchyma.

Clinical insight

The term contusion is not synonymous with laceration. A cerebral laceration is a specific type of injury in which there is tearing of the brain parenchyma.

Key facts

Contusions are a common finding in patients with traumatic brain injury. They are described as either coup or contrecoup.

- Coup contusions arise at the area of brain directly below the site of impact with an object
- Contrecoup contusions occur at the diametrically opposite side of the brain; they are the consequence of the brain impacting the adjacent skull as the patient rapidly decelerates
- Contusions vary in size and severity of clinical consequences. Severe contusions can cause oedema, mass effect and increased intracranial pressure (see section 3.6). Contusions may extend out of the parenchyma and into the subdural space to become what is termed a burst lobe
- Over the 24–48 hours following injury, the brain parenchyma surrounding a contusion may become increasingly oedematous and start to swell. This is known as the blossoming of the contusion

Imaging findings

CT Haemorrhagic contusions appear as hyperdensities that vary in location and size. They can occur at any site, but are most commonly located in the frontal lobe (**Figure 4.11**) and temporal lobe. Contusions can be large or small (petechial).

It is important to search for contrecoup contusions (**Figure 4.12**) because these are common.

Oedema may surround contusions; it appears hypodense. Follow-up imaging some days after the injury occurred may show worsening (blossoming) of contusions.

MRI This is more sensitive than CT for the detection of contusions. It can be used as a second-line investigation if CT fails to reveal suspected injury.

Management

Management of cerebral contusions depends on the neurological status of the patient. Smaller contusions in a neurologically intact patient are usually managed conservatively. However, patients with large contusions (associated with mass effect) and

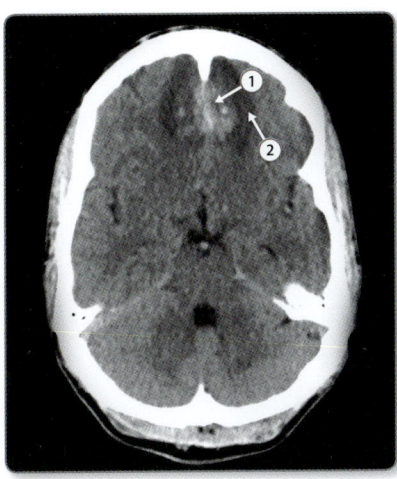

Figure 4.11 Axial CT scan showing bilateral frontal contusions. ① Haemorrhagic contusions, ② oedema.

a depressed conscious level usually require invasive intracranial pressure monitoring in intensive care.

4.7 Diffuse axonal injury

Diffuse axonal injury is an injury to the white matter caused by acceleration–deceleration or rotational forces. High-speed road traffic accidents are the most common cause.

Key facts
- Diffuse axonal injury is caused by shearing forces that most commonly affect the boundary between grey and white matter
- The corpus callosum and brainstem are common locations for diffuse axonal injury to occur
- Diffuse axonal injury can lead to chronic disorders of consciousness

Imaging findings
Diffuse axonal injury can be a subtle finding on neuroimaging. It may initially be overlooked in multiple intracranial injuries.

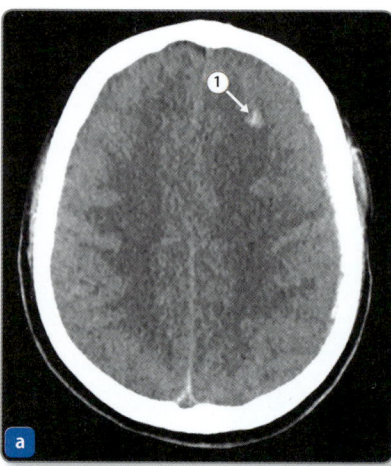

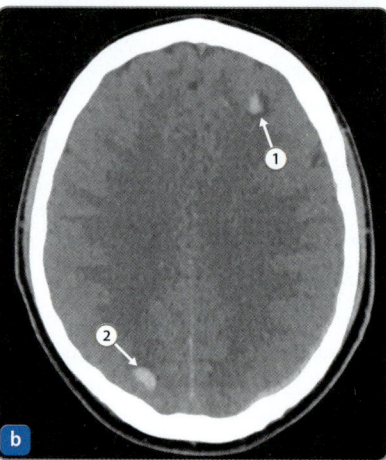

Figure 4.12 Axial CT scans in a case of traumatic brain injury caused by frontal impact. (a) Initial scan. (b) Scan obtained 24 hours after the injury, showing evolving contusions. ① Left frontal coup contusion, ② right occipital contrecoup contusion.

CT The appearance of diffuse axonal injury varies depending on its extent and whether or not the lesion is haemorrhagic. Haemorrhagic diffuse axonal injury appears hyperdense, whereas non-haemorrhagic diffuse axonal injury appears hypodense. CT is often insufficient for the detection of diffuse axonal injury.

MRI This is a more sensitive imaging modality than CT for the detection of diffuse axonal injury, because of the high spatial resolution it provides. Advanced MRI modalities, including magnetic resonance spectroscopy and diffusion-weighted imaging, are increasingly used in the investigation of diffuse axonal injury.

Management
Diffuse axonal injury has a poor prognosis. Survivors with severe diffuse axonal injury may be left in a chronic disorder of consciousness (a vegetative state). The mainstay of management is prevention of secondary brain injury.

Cerebrovascular disease

The term cerebrovascular disease encompasses pathologies of the blood vessels supplying the brain. The most common of these conditions is stroke.

Stroke is an acute neurological deficit, lasting at least 24 hours, caused by damage to part of the brain as a result of either interruption of blood flow or bleeding. It is a medical emergency. Patients presenting to the emergency department with suspected stroke require urgent assessment and treatment, and admission to an acute stroke unit for specialist treatment.

Other types of cerebrovascular disease include subarachnoid haemorrhage, arteriovenous malformation, carotid and vertebral artery dissection and dural venous sinus thrombosis.

5.1 Clinical scenario

Partial anterior circulation stroke

Presentation

A 70-year-old woman is brought to the emergency department. Her husband had suddenly noticed drooping on the left side of her face. Her left arm and leg had become weak. The husband had phoned an ambulance, and the patient arrived at the hospital about 30 minutes later. Clinical examination confirms left-sided weakness and reveals a left homonymous hemianopia (visual field defect). No other signs are detected, and there is no higher cerebral dysfunction. An urgent CT brain scan is carried out.

Initial interpretation

The patient's symptoms are consistent with stroke. The symptoms and signs meet the Oxford (Bamford) criteria for a diagnosis of partial anterior circulation stroke (**Table 5.1**). The left-sided weakness and visual field defect indicates that the right cerebral hemisphere is affected.

Type of stroke	Criteria
Total anterior circulation stroke	All three of the following: • Contralateral weakness or sensory loss of arm, leg or face • Contralateral homonymous hemianopia • Higher cerebral dysfunction
Partial anterior circulation stroke	Any two of the three features listed above
Lacunar stroke	One of: • Contralateral pure motor deficit • Contralateral pure sensory deficit • Ataxic hemiparesis
Posterior circulation stroke	One of: • Cerebellar dysfunction • Ipsilateral cranial nerve palsy • Isolated homonymous hemianopia • Bilateral motor or sensory deficit

Table 5.1 Oxford (Bamford) classification of stroke

Imaging findings

The CT head acquired on admission does not reveal any abnormalities, despite the presentation. However, a repeat scan taken 24 hours later reveals marked hypodensity of brain in the territory of the right middle cerebral artery (**Figure 5.1**).

Diagnosis

The symptoms and signs, along with the CT findings, support a diagnosis of a partial anterior circulation stroke.

Management

Because the clinical diagnosis is convincing, the patient has presented to hospital quickly, and the CT does not show haemorrhage, urgent intravenous thrombolysis or mechanical thrombectomy is warranted.

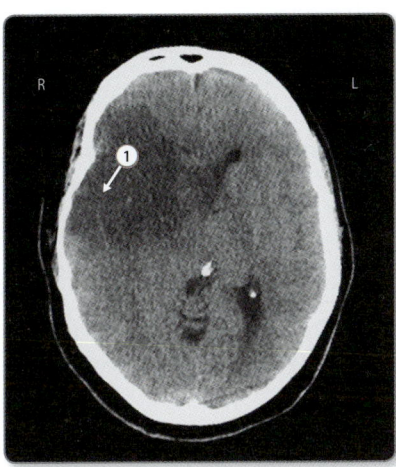

Figure 5.1 Axial CT scan (without contrast), obtained 24 hours after symptom onset. ① Large middle cerebral infarct, visible as an extensive hypodense area.

5.2 Ischaemic stroke and transient ischaemic attack

Ischaemic stroke is caused by interruption of blood supply to the brain, which if prolonged, results in infarction (death of tissue). The usual cause is acute arterial obstruction secondary to either localised thrombus formation or cardioembolism. About 85% of strokes are ischaemic.

A transient ischaemic attack ('mini-stroke') presents in the same way as a stroke but resolves in less than 24 hours. It is caused by temporary disruption of blood supply to the brain, and is not usually associated with identifiable infarct on imaging.

Careful history and examination will indicate the location of the lesion in suspected ischaemic stroke. However, an urgent CT scan is required before treatment for ischaemic stroke can be given, because it is essential to first exclude haemorrhagic stroke. This is because thrombolytic therapy, which is used to treat ischaemic stroke, would be catastrophic, worsening a haemorrhagic stroke.

Key facts

In clinical practice, ischaemic stroke is classified according to the Oxford (Bamford) system (see **Table 5.1**), which is based on the vessels affected.

- The anterior circulation is supplied by the internal carotid arteries, and supplies the anterior and middle cerebral arteries
- The perforating arteries of the anterior and middle cerebral arteries are perpendicular branches that supply the deep subcortical stuctures (e.g. basal ganglia and internal capsule). Occlusion of the vessels results in a lacunar stroke
- The posterior circulation is supplied by the vertebral arteries, and supplies the basilar artery, the cerebellar arteries and the posterior cerebral arteries

Imaging findings

Although the clinical symptoms and signs of stroke have a sudden onset, the imaging findings are relatively slow to evolve.

CT This is the first-line imaging modality in the diagnosis of stroke. Image acquisition is faster than with MRI, and CT is more readily available than MRI in most hospitals. Furthermore, CT is usually better tolerated by unwell, confused and claustrophobic patients.

Within hours of onset of stroke, the following features become apparent on CT.

- A hypodense (often wedge-shaped) region within the white matter and overlying cortex (see **Figure 5.1**)
- Loss of distinction between grey and white matter
- Loss of visualisation of the insular ribbon or other affected cortex
- Loss of differentiation of the basal ganglia
- Cytotoxic oedema within affected brain
- Hyperdense artery sign, commonly affecting the middle cerebral artery (**Figure 5.2**)

In ischaemic stroke, the CT scan commonly appears normal for the first few hours after symptom onset. Therefore, CT angiography or CT perfusion (**Figure 5.3**), or both, are increasingly being used in the acute management of ischaemic stroke to improve early diagnostic accuracy and to inform treatment decisions.

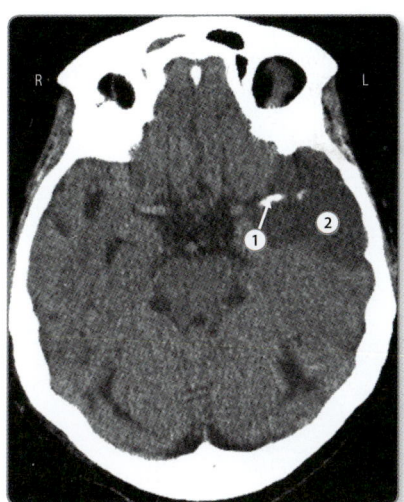

Figure 5.2 Axial CT scan (without contrast), showing ① a hyperdense left middle cerebral artery (consistent with thrombus) and ② resulting left middle cerebral artery infarct.

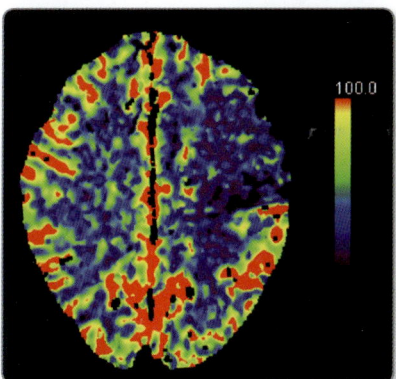

Figure 5.3 CT perfusion scan showing a deficit in cerebral blood flow in the left middle cerebral artery territory.

'Malignant' middle cerebral artery infarction is a consequence of complete occlusion of the middle cerebral artery. It usually occurs in younger patients without pre-existing brain atrophy, who therefore have very little intracranial space in which to accommodate swelling. Massive infarction with oedematous

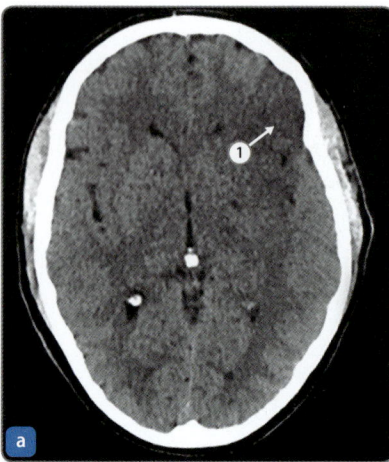

Figure 5.4 Axial CT scans (without contrast), showing malignant middle cerebral artery infarction. (a) First presentation shows a left middle cerebral artery infarct ①. (b) Repeat imaging shows extensive oedema ② and midline shift. (c) Postoperative imaging (several months later) shows absence of the skull and decompression of the brain. *Continues opposite*

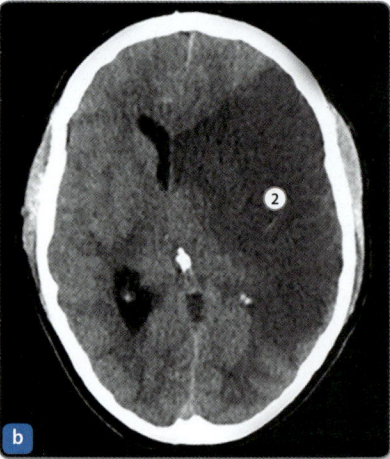

swelling results in increased intracranial pressure (**Figure 5.4**), which can be fatal.

MRI This imaging modality is less commonly used in the management of acute stroke, primarily for technical and logistic reasons. However, diffusion-weighted MRI can reveal acute ischaemic

Figure 5.4 Continued.

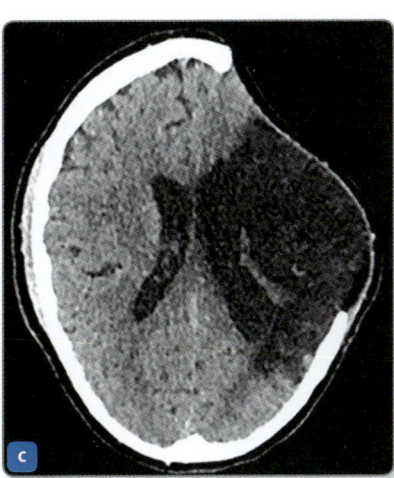

changes, apparent as increased diffusion-weighted signal with corresponding reduced apparent diffusion coefficient, within minutes of symptom onset (**Figure 5.5**). When compared to perfusion-weighted imaging, it is often possible to estimate the time of stroke onset and to speculate on the reversibility of the ischaemic lesion. Diffusion-weighted imaging and T2–FLAIR mismatch can also be used to estimate the time of stroke onset.

After a few hours, the ischaemic lesion may be visible as a region of hypointensity on T1-weighted MRI, and as a region of hyperintensity on T2-weighted MRI. These changes occur about the same time that brain changes start to become visible on CT. The appearance of infarct on MRI, as well as on CT, changes over the following weeks as the oedema resolves and injured brain tissue undergoes gliosis (scarring of the brain).

In a transient ischaemic attack, diffusion-weighted imaging should be carried out to investigate for ischaemic lesions (unless contraindicated). Diffusion-weighted imaging is far more sensitive than CT for the detection of small-volume ischaemic lesions.

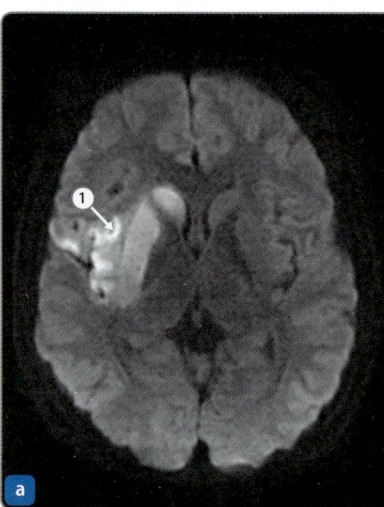

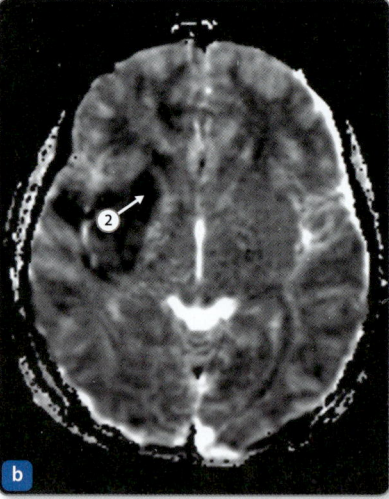

Figure 5.5 Axial MRI scans obtained within a few hours of development of symptoms and signs of stroke. (a) Diffusion-weighted imaging (DWI). (b) Apparent diffusion coefficient (ADC) imaging. The high signal on DWI ① and low signal on ADC imaging ② in the right middle cerebral artery territory in this context are consistent with recent infarction.

US All patients who have experienced a transient ischaemic attack, and some stroke patients, undergo US imaging of the carotid arteries as soon as possible after symptom onset. This is done to identify any potentially treatable arterial stenosis.

Management

All patients receive antiplatelet therapy after ischaemic stoke. Provided there are no contraindications and provided the interval between the stroke and presentation for treatment is less than 4.5 or 6 hours, respectively, patients receive either intravenous thrombolysis (using tissue plasminogen) activator or mechanical thrombectomy.

After these acute treatments, the main components of management are rehabilitation, identification of risk factors, and prevention of recurrence.

Malignant middle cerebral artery infarction requires referral to a neurosurgeon. Clinical trials have shown that decompressive craniectomy significantly improves survival in patients under the age of 60.

5.3 Haemorrhagic stroke: introduction

About 15% of strokes are haemorrhagic, caused by bleeding into or around the brain. There are two categories of haemorrhagic stroke:

- **Parenchymal brain haemorrhage** (also called intraparenchymal haemorrhage, and intracerebral haemorrhage or stroke), in which there is bleeding into the parenchyma of the brain: roughly two-thirds of haemorrhagic strokes
- **Subarachnoid haemorrhage** (SAH), in which there is bleeding into the subarachnoid space: roughly one-third of haemorrhagic strokes

The clinical manifestations and management are very distinct for these two types, so they are each discussed in a separate section below.

5.4 Parenchymal brain haemorrhage

In parenchymal brain haemorrhage there is bleeding into the parenchyma of the brain (hence the synonym intraparenchymal brain haemorrhage). About 15% of strokes are caused by parenchymal brain haemorrhage.

Key facts

- The main risk factor for primary parenchymal brain haemorrhage is hypertension
- Secondary parenchymal brain haemorrhage can be caused by a vascular abnormality (amyloid angiopathy, arteriovenous malformation, aneurysm or transformation of an arterial or venous infarction), trauma, brain tumour, drug misuse (cocaine can cause a sudden spike in blood pressure), bleeding disorders and use of anticoagulants
- Patients with hypertension typically bleed from the small perforating branches of the lenticulostriate arteries that supply the basal ganglia and internal capsule; these haemorrhages are called 'deep bleeds'

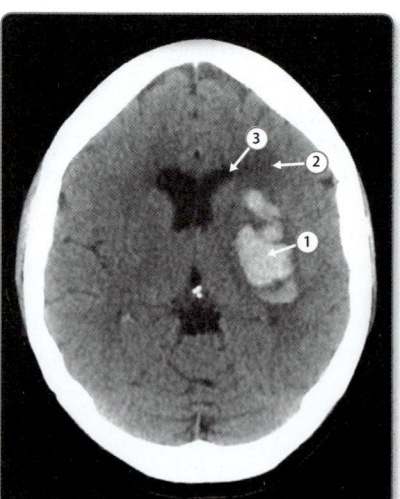

Figure 5.6 Axial CT scan from a patient with acute parenchymal brain haemorrhage. ① Intraparenchymal haematoma in the left basal ganglia, ② surrounding oedema, ③ local mass effect (effacement of the left lateral ventricle).

- Symptoms and signs of parenchymal brain haemorrhage include loss of consciousness, headache, nausea, vomiting, weakness, visual field loss and seizures

Imaging findings

CT This is the primary modality of choice in suspected parenchymal brain haemorrhage. Acute haemorrhage is visible as a hyperdense lesion on CT (**Figure 5.6**).

Although ruptured aneurysms usually bleed into the cerebrospinal fluid–filled subarachnoid space surrounding the brain (see Section 5.6), they can also bleed directly into the brain parenchyma. In the absence of an identifiable cause for bleeding, CT angiography or digital subtraction angiography may be carried out to assess for an underlying vascular abnormality.

Signs of increased intracranial pressure (see section 3.6) are sought. These are often associated with a rapid deterioration in the patient's condition, necessitating changes in clinical management.

MRI This is not typically used in the acute period of parenchymal brain haemorrhage. However, it may be used to investigate for underlying vascular abnormalities or tumour once the original haemorrhage has dissipated.

Management

Most parenchymal brain haemorrhages are managed conservatively, although surgery may be required in cases of obstructive hydrocephalus or deteriorating consciousness. Any underlying vascular abnormality present, such as an aneurysm or arteriovenous malformation, is treated accordingly.

5.5 Clinical scenario

Subarachnoid haemorrhage

Presentation

A 45-year-old woman presents to the emergency department after developing a severe occipital headache. The headache came on suddenly during a game of tennis, and is the worst she has ever had. On clinical examination, she has neck stiffness and photophobia. No other neurological deficits are detected, and her Glasgow Coma Scale (GCS) score is 15.

Initial interpretation

From the history and examination, this is a classic presentation of subarachnoid haemorrhage. An urgent CT scan is requested.

Imaging findings

The CT scan reveals hyperdensity within the basal cisterns and the lateral sulci (**Figure 5.7**).

Diagnosis

The CT scan confirms subarachnoid haemorrhage. The larger collection of blood in the right lateral sulcus raises the suspicion of aneurysm of the right middle cerebral artery.

Management

The patient is transferred to the neurosurgical department for further investigation and treatment. She is given analgesia, fluids and nimodipine pending further specialist imaging (usually CT angiography or digital subtraction angiography).

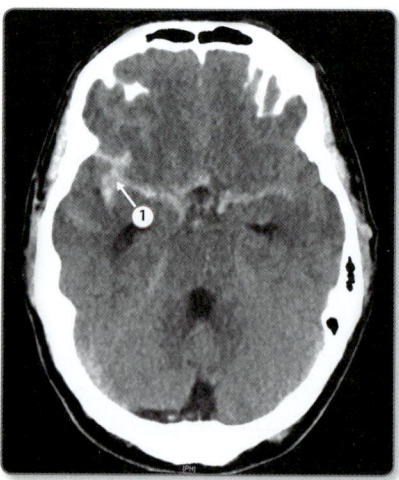

Figure 5.7 Axial CT scan (without contrast) from a patient with subarachnoid haemorrhage. ① Hyperdensity within the subarachnoid space, most prominent in the right lateral sulcus.

5.6 Subarachnoid haemorrhage

Subarachnoid haemorrhage describes the presence of blood within the subarachnoid space.

Key facts

- The most common cause of subarachnoid haemorrhage is trauma. In non-traumatic (or 'spontaneous') cases, 85% are due to rupture of a saccular (berry) aneurysm. Other spontaneous causes include arteriovenous malformation, vasculitis or arterial dissection
- The classic symptoms and signs of non-traumatic subarachnoid haemorrhage are a sudden 'thunderclap' headache, neck stiffness, photophobia, and in severe cases, reduced consciousness
- Subarachnoid haemorrhage is classified using the World Federation of Neurosurgical Societies grading scale (**Table 5.2**), which is based on GCS score and focal neurological deficit
- Complications of subarachnoid haemorrhage include electrolyte disturbance, hydrocephalus, seizures and vasospasm leading to delayed cerebral ischaemia and infarction
- Aneurysmal subarachnoid haemorrhage is occasionally complicated by rebleeding

Imaging findings

CT The first-line investigation in suspected subarachnoid haemorrhage is non-contrast CT (see **Figure 5.7**). If carried

Grade	Glasgow Coma Scale score	Focal neurological deficit
1	15	Absent
2	13 or 14	Absent
3	13 or 14	Present
4	7–12	Present or absent
5	3–6	Present or absent

Table 5.2 World Federation of Neurosurgical Societies grading scale for subarachnoid haemorrhage

Clinical insight

A posterior communicating artery aneurysm can cause a third cranial nerve palsy, because of the proximity of the two structures. This results in ipsilateral 'down and out' deviation of the eye, ptosis (drooping eyelid) and pupillary dilation.

out within 24 hours of onset, acute haemorrhage (hyperdensity) is visible in the subarachnoid space in 95% of cases. However, the detection rate decreases over time, as the blood becomes less dense: CT carried out 7 days after onset of symptoms is very unlikely to provide radiological evidence of subarachnoid haemorrhage.

If there are no features of subarachnoid haemorrhage on CT but clinical suspicion remains high, lumbar puncture is required to exclude the presence of blood products within the cerebrospinal fluid (**Figure 5.8**). If the lumbar puncture reveals blood products, then subarachnoid haemorrhage is confirmed and CT angiography or digital subtraction angiography (DSA) is used to search for a vascular cause.

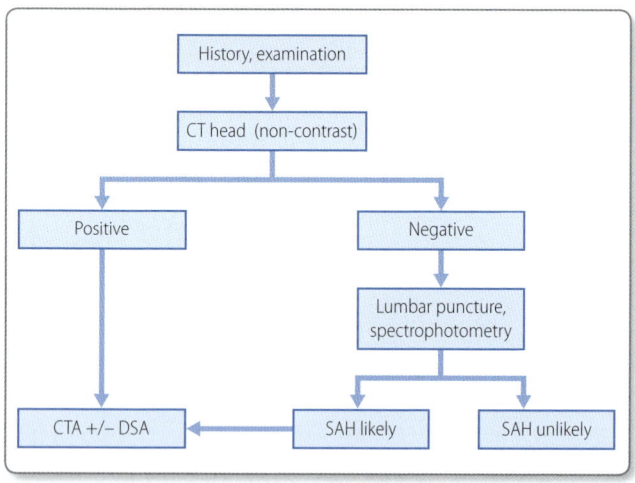

Figure 5.8 Investigation pathway in non-traumatic subarachnoid haemorrhage (SAH). DSA, digital subtraction angiography; CTA, CT angiography.

Subarachnoid blood typically accumulates in the basal cisterns, lateral sulci (Sylvian fissures), cerebral sulci and ventricles. The modified Fisher grading scale is used to allocate a score based on the thickness of the blood and the presence of blood in the ventricles (**Table 5.3**). Intraventricular blood and hydrocephalus are poor prognostic signs; the patient's condition may deteriorate rapidly unless an external ventricular drain is inserted to relieve increased intracranial pressure.

An underlying aneurysm or other vascular malformation is rarely identifiable on non-contrast CT. However, the site of maximal haemorrhage suggests, but does not prove, the location of origin of the bleed.

CT angiography and digital subtraction angiography Both CT angiography (**Figure 5.9**) and digital subtraction angiography (**Figure 5.10**) are used to search for aneurysms and other vascular malformations.

MRI Neither MRI nor magnetic resonance angiography (MRA) are used routinely for the management of acute subarachnoid haemorrhage. However, MRA is commonly used for follow-up of patients who have received treatment for an aneurysm. MRA spares them from repeated irradiation from CT and the risks associated with traditional angiography; furthermore, it overcomes the problem that metallic devices such as clips and coils used for treating aneurysm create significant imaging artefact on CT. Nowadays, most coils and clips used in aneurysmal repair are not ferromagnetic, but before MRI or MRA follow up it is

Grade	Subarachnoid haemorrhage	Intraventricular haemorrhage
0	Absent	Absent
1	Thin (< 1 mm deep)	Absent
2	Thin (< 1 mm deep)	Present
3	Thick (> 1 mm deep)	Absent
4	Thick (> 1 mm deep)	Present

Table 5.3 The modified Fisher grading scale for subarachnoid haemorrhage

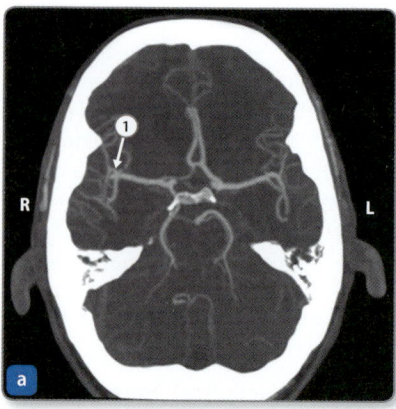

Figure 5.9 CT angiograms: (a) axial section and (b) three-dimensional reconstruction. ① Aneurysm at the right middle cerebral artery bifurcation. The right–left orientation is different in the reconstructed image.

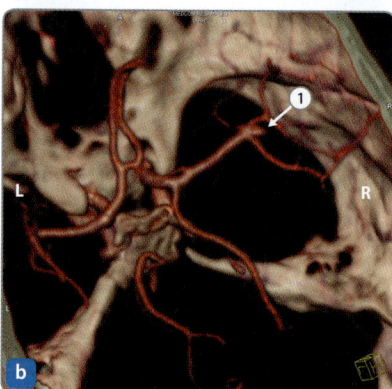

essential to rule out the presence of ferrous materials, especially if the aneurysm was treated over 10 years ago.

Management

Subarachnoid haemorrhage requires emergency management. Patients whose condition is unstable require admission to an intensive care unit. Ruptured aneurysms are treated as soon as possible after detection to prevent a re-bleed. This is done either with endovascular coiling (**Figure 5.11**) by an interventional

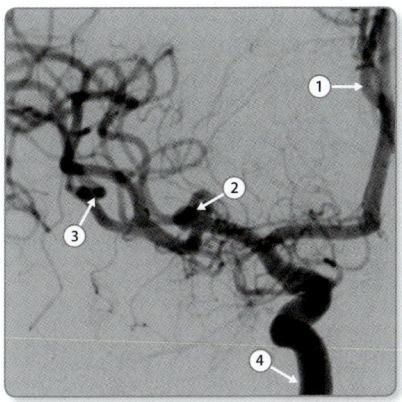

Figure 5.10
Anteroposterior digital subtraction angiogram of the right internal carotid artery and its major branches. ① Anterior cerebral artery, ② right middle cerebral artery aneurysm, ③ branches of the middle cerebral artery, ④ right internal carotid artery.

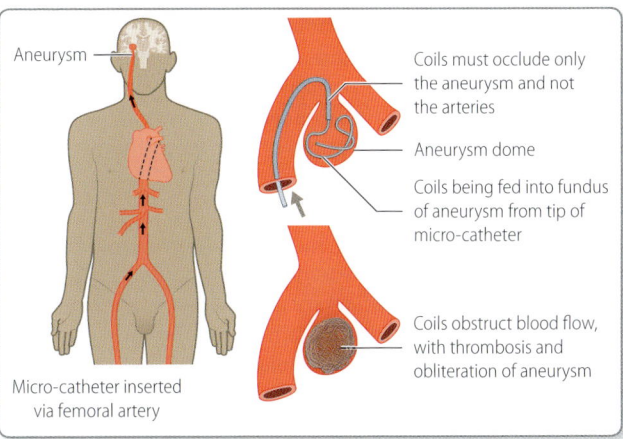

Aneurysm

Coils must occlude only the aneurysm and not the arteries

Aneurysm dome

Coils being fed into fundus of aneurysm from tip of micro-catheter

Coils obstruct blood flow, with thrombosis and obliteration of aneurysm

Micro-catheter inserted via femoral artery

Figure 5.11 Endovascular coiling, a minimally invasive technique commonly used to treat aneurysms and other neurovascular conditions. In the UK, it is carried out by interventional neuroradiologists. The vascular system is accessed, usually via the femoral artery, and a catheter is passed under radiographic guidance into the neurovascular system. Platinum coils are used to occlude the aneurysm.

neuroradiologist or, less commonly, by a neurosurgeon (clipping). Nimodipine, a selective calcium channel blocker that prevents vasospasm, is given to reduce the risk of delayed cerebral ischaemia and infarction.

5.7 Arteriovenous malformation

An arteriovenous malformation is an abnormal, disorganised tangle of blood vessels. They can be found anywhere in the body, including in the brain.

Key facts

- Arteriovenous malformations are mostly congenital, but can also be acquired
- An arteriovenous malformation has one or several of both feeding arteries and draining veins
- The nidus is the transition point between the feeding artery and the draining vein; there are no intervening capillaries
- Arteriovenous malformations may be asymptomatic or present clinically with focal neurological deficits, seizures or parenchymal or subarachnoid brain haemorrhage

Imaging findings

CT An arteriovenous malformation is visible on CT as a disorganised, heterogeneous but predominantly hyperdense mass (**Figure 5.12a**). There are often flecks of calcification (of similar density to the skull), and the adjacent brain may show oedema. On CT angiography, the underlying vascular nature is much more apparent, sometimes described as a 'bag of worms' (**Figure 5.13a**).

MRI T2-weighted MRI shows multiple serpiginous flow voids (**Figure 5.12b**). Evidence of haemorrhage may also be visible, particularly on haem-sensitive sequences, T2* or susceptibility-weighted imaging.

Digital subtraction angiography An arteriovenous malformation can be viewed in further detail on a digital subtraction angiogram. The feeding and draining vessels are often more apparent, and the temporal nature of blood flow through the arteriovenous malformation more easily appreciated (**Figure 5.13b**).

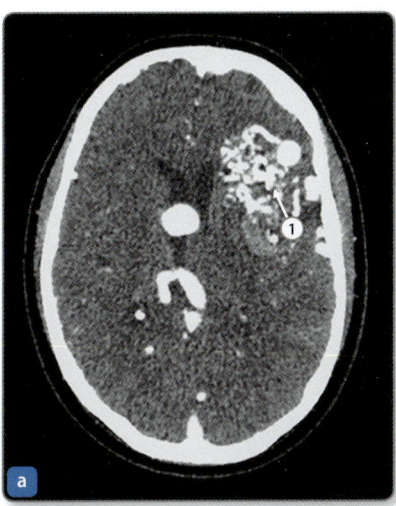

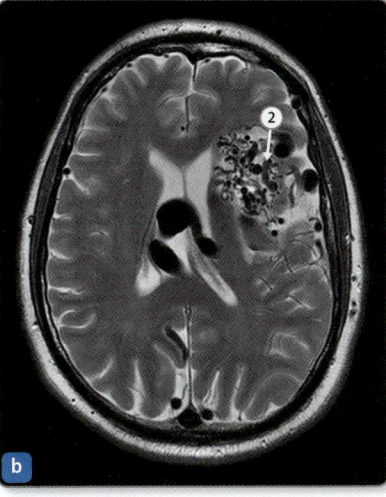

Figure 5.12 (a) Axial CT scan (post-contrast) and (b) axial T2-weighted MRI scan showing a left frontotemporal arteriovenous malformation. ① Hyperdense area with irregular, serpiginous structures, ② multiple flow voids.

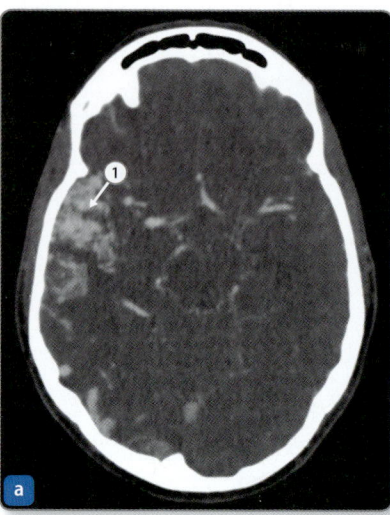

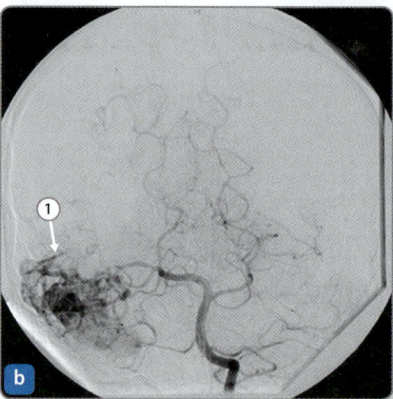

Figure 5.13 Axial CT angiogram (a) and anteroposterior digital subtraction angiogram (b) showing a right temporal arteriovenous malformation ①.

Management

Arteriovenous malformations are managed with one or a combination of the following: conservative management, neurosurgery (surgical excision), interventional neuroradiology (endovascular embolisation of both feeding arteries and draining veins) or radiation therapy.

5.8 Carotid and vertebral artery dissection

An arterial dissection is a flap-like tear in the intimal lining of an artery, which allows blood to enter the arterial wall and form a false lumen. This process leads to narrowing or occlusion of the true lumen. Subsequent thrombus formation in the true arterial lumen can compound the problem, reducing arterial flow further. Therefore, arterial dissection can cause ischaemic stroke.

Key facts

- Dissection can be caused by trauma (direct or deceleration injury) or arise spontaneously in individuals with connective tissue disease (e.g. Marfan's or Ehlers–Danlos syndrome); in some instances, however, no cause is identified
- Symptoms include headache, neck pain and features of stroke
- An ipsilateral oculosympathetic palsy (Horner's syndrome) may develop in internal carotid artery dissection in which sympathetic nerves in the arterial wall are disturbed
- Vertebral dissection typically arises at the C1–C2 level, whereas internal carotid dissection typically arises at the C3–C4 level; dissection flaps are often longitudinally extensive from their point of origin

Imaging findings

CT angiography Visualisation of the arterial supply to the brain by CT angiography reveals arterial narrowing or occlusion (**Figure 5.14a**). Residual flow within an affected arterial segment often has a tapered, spiral appearance. CT angiography may include imaging of the brain, allowing a search for secondary infarction.

MRI Use of a fat-saturated T1-weighted sequence may better visualise haematoma in the wall of the artery. MRI is

> ### Clinical insight
>
> Features of oculosympathetic palsy (Horner's syndrome) include ipsilateral ptosis (drooping of the eyelid), miosis (constricted pupil) and anhidrosis (reduced sweating).

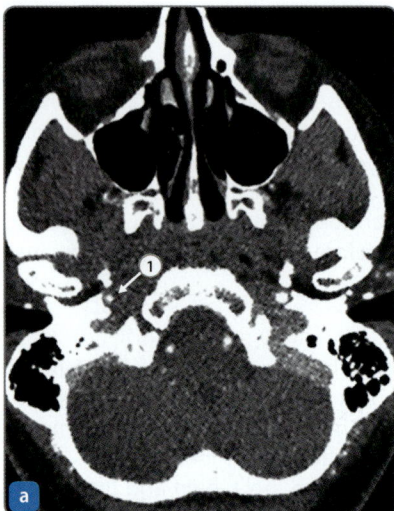

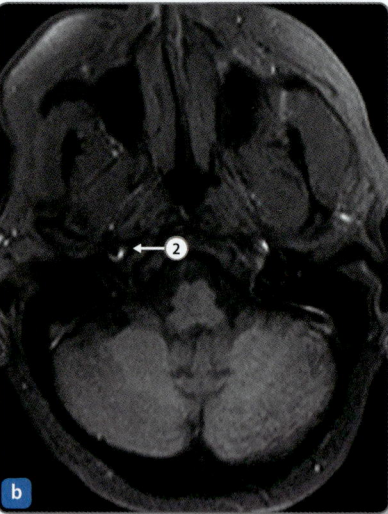

Figure 5.14 Axial CT angiogram (a) and axial T1-weighted MRI scan (fat-saturated) (b) showing dissection of the right internal carotid artery. ① Narrowing of the lumen of the right internal carotid artery compared with that of the left internal carotid artery. ② The dissection, visible as a crescenteric area of high signal.

also more sensitive for detecting secondary infarct in the brain (**Figure 5.14b**).

Management
Arterial dissection is mostly managed by anticoagulation and lifestyle modification. Arterial stenting is considered when medical management has failed.

5.9 Dural venous sinus thrombosis

Dural venous sinus thrombosis is difficult to diagnose and there are several aetiologies. Thrombosis can occur in any part of the intracranial venous system, and can lead to cerebral infarction and haemorrhage.

Key facts
- The most common risk factors for dural venous sinus thrombosis are trauma, infection (e.g. in mastoiditis), chronic inflammatory disease (e.g. inflammatory bowel disease), cancer, clotting disorders or use of certain drugs (e.g. the combined oral contraceptive pill)
- The clinical features of dural venous sinus thrombosis are variable but include headache, confusion and visual disturbances. Onset of symptoms is usually not sudden; they may develop or worsen over several days. Progression of the condition leads to seizures, drowsiness and coma

Imaging findings

CT   The changes on CT may be subtle. On unenhanced CT, the venous sinuses are not typically hyperdense unless thrombosed. Using CT with contrast (venous phase), DVST may be identified as filling defects within the venous sinuses, e.g. dural venous sinus thrombosis within the sagittal sinus may exhibit the empty delta sign (clot identified as a triangular filling deficit).

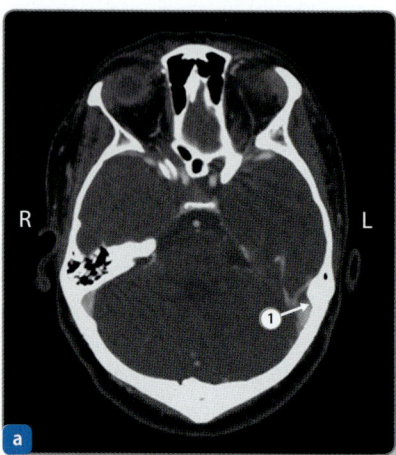

Figure 5.15 (a) Axial CT venogram in a patient with dural venous sinus thrombosis. (1) Hypodense filling defect in the left transverse sinus. (b) Magnetic resonance venogram (three-dimensional reconstruction) in a different patient. (2) Absent flow in the right transverse sinus. (3) Normal filling of the left transverse sinus.

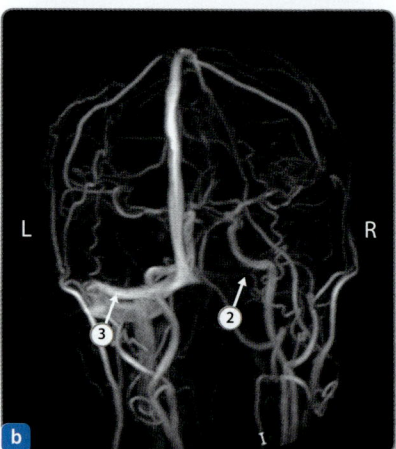

CT venography A CT venogram shows failure of normal filling of sinuses, filling defects (**Figure 5.15a**), or both. CT also allows investigation for secondary infarction and haemorrhage. Unlike stroke caused by arterial occlusion, cerebral infarction in dural venous sinus thrombosis is not confined to arterial vascular territories.

MRI In dural venous sinus thrombosis, lack of flow void is most apparent on T2-weighted imaging. This filling defect may appear hyperintense on T1-weighted imaging if the thrombus is acute or subacute. Magnetic resonance venography may also be used; loss of signal indicates a filling defect (**Figure 5.15b**).

Management
Dural venous sinus thrombosis is managed by lifestyle modification and anticoagulation therapy. If haemorrhage is found on imaging, the benefits and risks of anticoagulation need to be considered.

Inflammatory disorders

Inflammation is the biological response to injury. Primary inflammatory brain diseases are due to maladaptive inflammation against the brain parenchyma (e.g. multiple sclerosis, neurosarcoidosis or encephalitis) or the blood vessels of the brain (CNS vasculitis).

6.1 Multiple sclerosis

Multiple sclerosis (MS) is an autoimmune disorder of the central nervous system (CNS). Acutely, it causes inflammation, manifesting as acute plaques. The inflammation progresses to demyelination (destruction of the myelin sheath) over time, resulting in chronic plaques.

Key facts
- In the UK, about 100,000 people currently have MS
- It is about twice as common in women, and usually presents between the ages of 20 and 40 years
- The presentation of MS varies, because inflammation and demyelination occur at different sites within the CNS, and therefore cause different neurological deficits. MS commonly presents with optic neuritis, sensory symptoms or motor symptoms, or a combination of these
- Progression of MS varies. Some patients experience few symptoms for many years. Others develop permanent neurological deficits resulting from axonal death. The classic pattern of MS progression is relapsing–remitting, with acute demyelination causing 'attacks' of symptoms, and healing resulting in their partial or complete relief
- Diagnosis of MS is based on clinical assessment, laboratory test results and MRI findings. The revised McDonald diagnostic criteria for MS require two or more lesions to be detected on MRI at different times (i.e. separate episodes of MS) and at different sites within the CNS

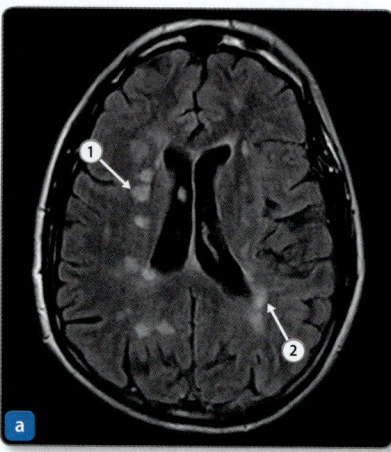

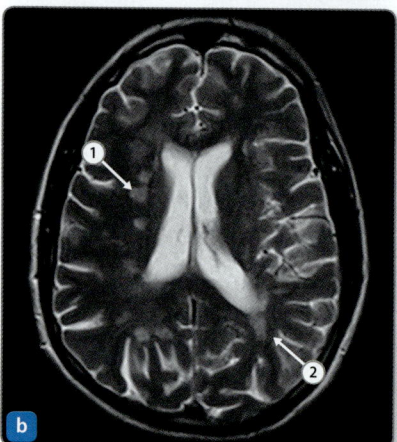

Figure 6.1 MRI scans of the brain of a patient with multiple sclerosis: (a) Axial, T2–FLAIR, (b) axial, T2-weighted and (c) sagittal, T2–FLAIR. ① Subcortical white matter lesions, ② periventricular white matter lesions, ③ 'Dawson's fingers'. *Continues opposite.*

- The differential diagnosis for MS includes vasculitis, neuro-sarcoidosis and neuromyelitis optica

Imaging findings

Diagnosis of MS is based primarily on clinical assessment, i.e. symptoms and signs. However, the results of imaging studies

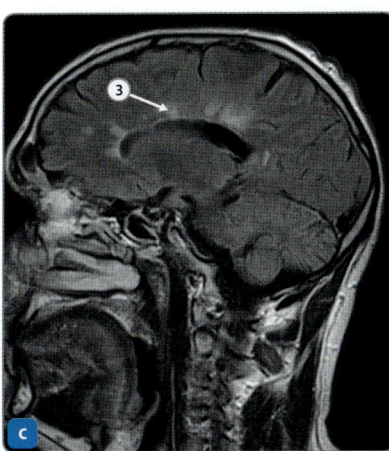

Figure 6.1 *Continued.*

and other tests (cerebrospinal fluid analysis and evoked potential testing) can strengthen the diagnosis or help exclude differential diagnoses.

CT The plaques of MS may appear as areas of hypodensity on CT. However, it is neither sensitive nor specific for MS; MRI is required.

MRI The plaques of MS are white matter lesions.

Like other white matter lesions, MS plaques appear hyperintense on T2-weighted MRI and T2–FLAIR (**Figure 6.1**). They appear isointense or hypointense on T1-weighted MRI.

Features on MRI that are more specific to MS are:

- Involvement of the corpus callosum, temporal lobes, periventricular region, brainstem, cerebellar peduncles, optic nerves and spinal cord (**Figure 6.2**)

> ## Clinical insight
>
> Features of MS can be incidental findings on neuroimaging, in cases of what is called radiologically isolated syndrome. Conversely, symptoms of MS may be present without evidence of MS on neuroimaging, in cases of clinically isolated syndrome. In both syndromes, MS may or may not progress.

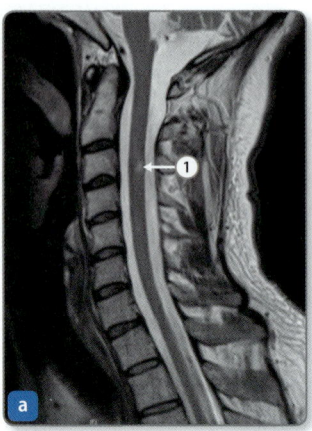
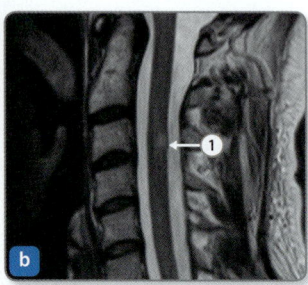

Figure 6.2 Sagittal T2-weighted MRI scan of the cervical spine, showing multiple sclerosis involving the spinal cord. ① High signal indicating a white matter cord lesion at the C3 level.

- Juxtacortical U-shaped lesions visible at the border between grey and white matter
- 'Dawson's fingers' (finger-like projections oriented perpendicular to the lateral ventricles)
- Contrast enhancement of acute lesions

Management

Multiple sclerosis is managed by neurologists. Patients are treated with immunosuppressive agents (e.g. steroids and monoclonal antibodies).

6.2 Sarcoidosis

Sarcoidosis is an inflammatory disease that affects multiple systems of the body. In this condition, granulomas, i.e. collections of inflammatory cells called macrophages, form within organs.

Sarcoidosis with CNS involvement is referred to as neurosarcoidoisis.

Key facts

- The clinical presentation of neurosarcoidosis is highly variable, and patients may be asymptomatic. Symptoms and signs may be specific to the CNS region (i.e focal neurological deficits) or non-specific (e.g. seizures or endocrine disturbance)
- Cranial nerve palsies are common; they are a consequence of involvement of the meninges at the skull base
- Neurosarcoidosis can mimic other conditions, including MS, vasculitis and tumour

Imaging findings

The most sensitive modality for assessment of neurosarcoidosis is MRI.

MRI White matter lesions are seen as patchy hypointensities on T1-weighted MRI, or hyperintensities on T2-weighted MRI or T2–FLAIR. These lesions tend to enhance with contrast (**Figure 6.3**).

Meningeal involvement is indicated by focal or widespread enhancement with contrast around the base of the brain, the

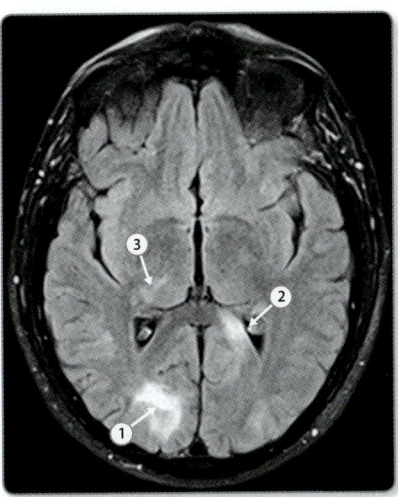

Figure 6.3 Axial MRI T2–FLAIR scan showing neurosarcoidosis. White matter lesions are present in the right occipital lobe ①, left corpus callosum ② and right thalamus ③.

circle of Willis or the perforating vessels (perivascular spaces). Meningeal involvement occasionally leads to hydrocephalus.

Management

Neurosarcoidosis is treated with steroids and immunosuppressive therapy.

Infections

Infections of the central nervous system can be bacterial, viral, fungal or caused by other rare agents (e.g. prion disease).

Bacterial infections, the focus of this chapter, are invariably life-threatening and require urgent assessment and treatment.

7.1 Clinical scenario

Cerebral abscess

Presentation

A 60-year-old, right-handed woman presents to the emergency department after developing progressive weakness in her right arm and right leg, and confusion, over the past 3 days. Her past medical history includes multiple myeloma, and she has recently completed a course of chemotherapy.

Examination confirms the weakness described as well as dysphasia. The patient has a temperature of 38.5°C. There are no other remarkable findings.

The emergency department doctor requests an urgent CT head and a septic screen as part of their investigations.

Initial interpretation

The neurological deficits suggest a left cerebral hemisphere lesion. The 3-day progression of the symptoms makes a vascular cause, such as stroke, less likely.

> ### Clinical insight
>
> **Meningitis** describes inflammation of the meninges. It can be specified as either **leptomeningitis** (inflammation of the leptomeninges, i.e. the arachnoid and pia mater) or **pachymeningitis** (inflammation of the dura mater). Infection, either bacterial or viral, is a common cause of meningitis.
>
> **Encephalitis** describes inflammation of the brain parenchyma. It is classified by the region affected; for example, **cerebritis** is inflammation of the cerebrum. Causes include viral or bacterial infection, and autoimmune disease.
>
> **Ventriculitis** describes inflammation of the ependymal layer that lines the ventricular system. Causes of ventriculitis include spreading infective meningitis or encephalitis, intraventricular haemorrhage or surgery (e.g. iatrogenic infection from a ventricular–peritoneal shunt or external ventricular drain).

The presence of fever in an immunocompromised patient raises the suspicion of infection. When accompanied by neurological symptoms, a neurological infection is suspected. If the fever is in response to a non-neurological infection (e.g. a urinary tract or chest infection), the history could be ascribed to a subdural haematoma or intra-axial mass, such as a primary or secondary brain tumour.

Imaging findings

The CT with contrast reveals a mass in the left temporal lobe (**Figure 7.1**). It is spherical, measures about 30 mm by 30 mm, is centrally hypodense and has a thin, regular enhancing rim. The surrounding hypodensity is compatible with oedema. There is midline shift and left ambient effacement caused by descending incisural herniation. Based on these CT findings, the differential diagnosis includes cerebral abscess, which would require urgent neurosurgical intervention. Therefore, an urgent MRI scan is requested to investigate further.

The MRI scan confirms a solitary mass (**Figure 7.2**). T1-weighted imaging shows a hypointense core with a congruous enhancing

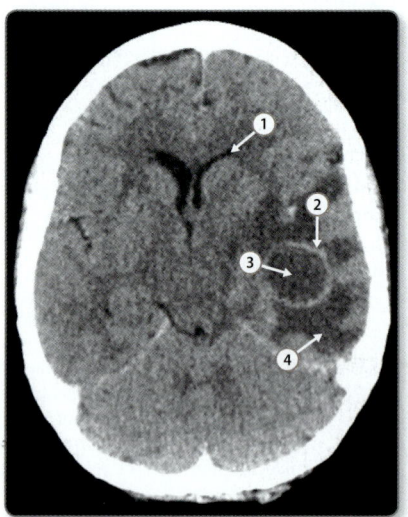

Figure 7.1 CT scan of the head (with contrast), showing a left temporal abscess. ① Mass effect with effacement of the frontal horn of the left lateral ventricle, ② rim-enhancing (hyperdense) effect on contrast, ③ hypodense abscess cavity, ④ vasogenic oedema.

rim (**Figure 7.2a**). T2-weighted imaging shows a hyperintense core with a congruous hypointense rim, and hyperintense surrounding parenchyma (**Figure 7.2b**). Restricted diffusion is visible as hyperintensity on the diffusion-weighted image.

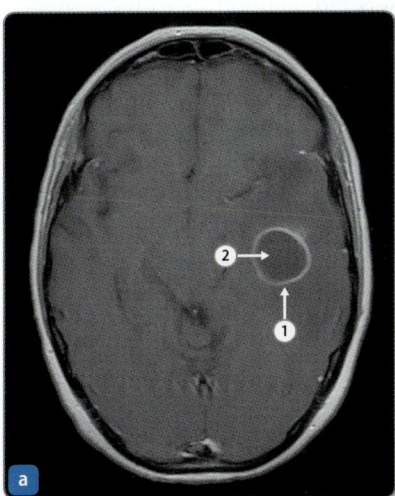

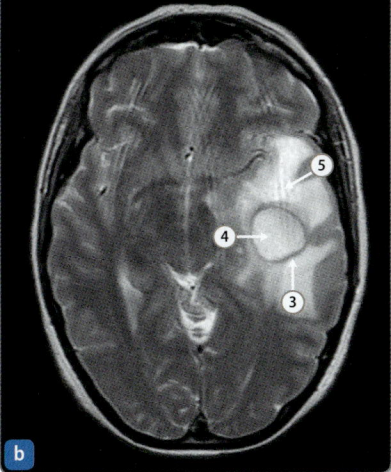

Figure 7.2 Axial MRI scans showing a left temporal abscess (same patient as in Figure 7.1): (a) T1-weighted (post contrast) and (b) T2-weighted. ① Rim-enhancing (hyperintense) effect, ② hypointense abscess cavity. ③ Hypointense rim, ④ hyperintense cavity, ⑤ hyperintense vasogenic oedema.

Subsequent CT of the chest, abdomen and pelvis shows no other lesions.

Diagnosis

A broad differential diagnosis is considered for a rim-enhancing, intra-axial mass. The restricted diffusion steers the diagnosis away from a tumour and towards a cerebral abscess. In this situation, chemotherapy has rendered the patient immunosuppressed and more susceptible to this condition.

7.2 Cerebral abscess

An abscess is a collection of pus that is contained within a capsule of inflammatory tissue. A cerebral abscess develops as a consequence of infection of the cerebrum (cerebritis) followed by formation of a capsule.

Key facts

- The main risk factors for cerebral abscess are: immunosuppression, bacterial endocarditis (e.g. in intravenous drug users), systemic sepsis, middle ear infection, dental infection and sinus infection
- The differential diagnosis of a cerebral abscess includes necrotic tumours (e.g. high-grade glioma or cerebral metastases), contusion, demyelination, resolving haematoma and old infarct

Imaging findings

CT Use of CT before and after administration of contrast allows identification of a rim-enhancing lesion (see **Figure 7.1**). The capsule is highly vascularised and enhances with contrast. The pus in the cavity within is not vascularised, and remains hypodense. The surrounding parenchyma is hypodense because of the presence of vasogenic oedema.

MRI This is the imaging modality of choice for cerebral abscess. It is more sensitive for the detection of this abnormality and its differentiation from other lesions (see **Figure 7.2**).

Post-contrast T1-weighted MRI shows a rim-enhancing (hyperintense) capsule and a hypointense cavity (see **Figure 7.2a**), similar to the CT appearance. T2-weighted MRI and T2–FLAIR show a variable appearance of the capsule; typically, there is hyperintensity of both the abscess cavity and the vasogenic oedema (see **Figure 7.2b**). The abscess cavity is visible as high intensity on a diffusion-weighted imaging sequence (**Figure 7.3**), owing to restricted diffusion.

Clinical insight

A well-known and useful mnemonic for considering the differential diagnosis of a rim-enhancing lesion is MAGICAL DR:

Metastasis

Abscess

Glioma (typically high-grade)

Infarct

Contusion

AIDS-related lesions

Lymphoma or lymphoproliferative disorders

Demyelination

Resolving haematoma

Management

Urgent referral to neurosurgery is required. Most are managed by drainage of the abscess, sampling for culture and sensitivity, and administration of a long course of intravenous

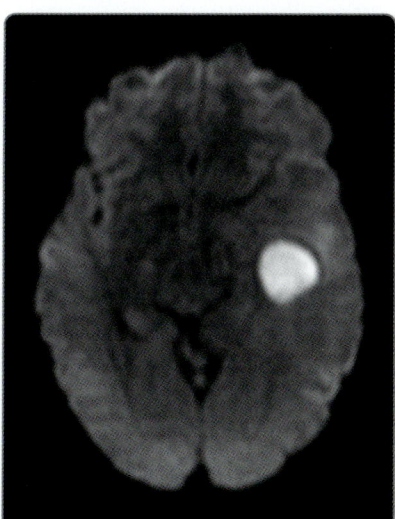

Figure 7.3 Diffusion-weighted MRI scan showing a left temporal abscess (same patient as in Figures 7.1 and 7.2). Restricted diffusion is visible as a region of hyperintensity showing the abscess cavity.

antibiotics. After acute management, the underlying cause is sought and risk factors are determined.

7.3 Subdural and extradural empyema

A subdural empyema is a collection of pus within the subdural space. Subdural empyemas account for around 20% of all intra-cranial infections. An extradural empyema is a collection of pus superficial to the dural meningeal layer. Extradural empyemas are less common than subdural empyemas.

Key facts
- Common causes of empyema are haematogenous spread of infection, paranasal (particularly frontal) sinusitis, mastoiditis and iatrogenic infection from previous surgery
- Patients with empyema typically present with fever, seizures, decreased consciousness or focal neurological deficit
- It occasionally leads to infection of the brain and give rise to a cerebral abscess

Imaging findings
CT Empyemas appear as extra-axial, crescenteric collections that are not confined by suture lines (**Figure 7.4**). Extradural empyemas appear as extra-axial, lentiform or bi-convex collections that are restricted by suture lines. Unlike subdural haematomas or epidural haematomas, respectively, empyemas will typically have a contrast enhancing border. A caveat is that some chronic subdural haematomas have thickened and calcified rims.

MRI Empyemas commonly appear hyperintense on T1-weighted MRI and hypointense on T2-weighted MRI. Typically, there is contrast enhancement of the empyema boundary. As with cerebral abscess, the empyema collection is likely to show restricted diffusion.

Management
As with cerebral abscess, empyema requires neurosurgical referral for drainage, sampling for culture and sensitivity, and administration of intravenous antibiotics.

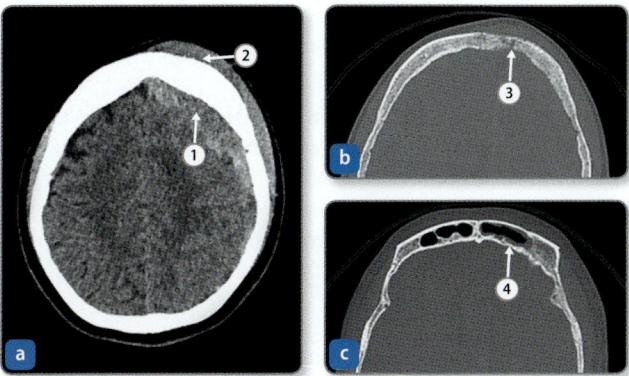

Figure 7.4 CT scans from a patient with subdural empyema: (a) unaltered window and (b and c) bone window. ① Subdural empyema, ② soft tissue infection, ③ osteomyelitis, ④ frontal sinus mucosal inflammation.

7.4 Spinal epidural abscess

A spinal epidural (less commonly termed 'extradural') abscess is a collection of pus within the extradural space.

Key facts

- The presentation of spinal epidural abscess is variable and often insidious. Clinical features include a combination of fever, back pain, nerve root pain, and neurological deficit according to the level of the lesion (e.g. motor deficit, sensory deficit, or bladder or bowel dysfunction or incontinence)
- Risk factors are local infection (e.g. from facet joint infection or discitis), systemic infection, intravenous drug use, immunosuppression, spinal trauma and surgery

Imaging findings

The imaging modality of choice is MRI with contrast, because CT is usually not sensitive enough to detect spinal epidural abscess. Spinal radiographs offer no appreciable benefit.

A scan of the whole spine is obtained to investigate the full extent of the abscess and to look for any skip lesions (discontiguous multilevel involvement).

MRI A spinal epidural abscess appears hypointense on T1-weighted MRI but enhances with contrast (**Figure 7.5**). It is hyperintense on T2-weighted MRI.

Spinal abscesses occur either anterior or posterior to the spinal cord. In specialist centres, spinal diffusion-weighted imaging is used to assess for restricted diffusion.

Management

Spinal epidural abscess is a neurosurgical emergency, because the expanding collection of pus will damage the spinal

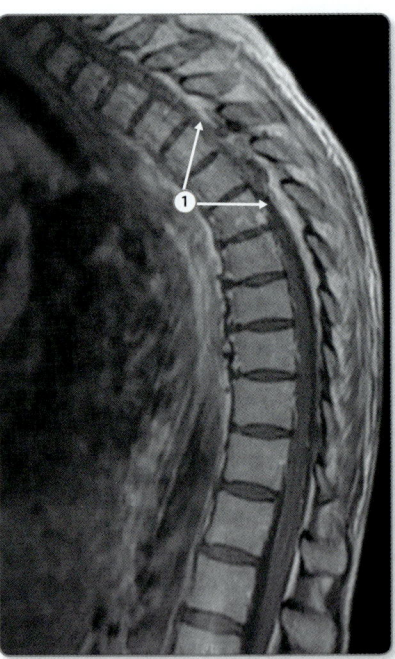

Figure 7.5 Sagittal T1-weighted MRI scan (post contrast) of the thoracic spine, showing spinal epidural (extradural) abscess ① extending from levels T2 to T9.

cord and spinal nerves by the processes of compression and inflammation. Surgical management includes decompression, washout and obtaining samples for culture. This is followed by administration of a long course of intravenous antibiotics.

Intracranial tumours

A tumour (or neoplasm) is an abnormal growth of tissue caused by uncontrolled cellular proliferation. A primary brain tumour is a tumour that has originated in the brain and resembles or is derived from cells of the nervous system. In the UK, this type of tumour has an annual incidence of 10 in 100,000 people. A secondary brain tumour – brain metastasis – is a tumour that has spread to the brain from its site of origin in another part of the body. Primary brain tumours are the most common solid tumours in children.

There are many types of brain tumour. They differ in their pathology, for example in terms of their benign (non-cancerous) or malignant (cancerous) nature, therefore outcomes, complications and prognosis vary greatly.

Spinal tumours are covered in Chapter 9.

8.1 Clinical scenario

Brain tumour

Presentation

A 40-year-old woman had attended her local optician with a headache. She wears glasses and thought that she needed a new prescription. However, her optician discovered 'worrying findings' during the eye test and advised her to go to the emergency department. The emergency department doctor learns from her history that she has experienced a 6-week, constant, progressively worsening and diffuse headache made worse by lying down or coughing. For the past 5 days, she has vomited after waking up in the morning.

Examination reveals no focal neurological deficits, but papilloedema is seen on fundoscopy. A CT head is requested by the emergency department doctor.

Initial interpretation

Headache of the nature described and associated with nausea is consistent with increased intracranial pressure. The time course indicates a slow-growing, space-occupying lesion.

Imaging findings

The CT scan shows a lesion in the right cerebral hemisphere, with associated mass effect and midline shift (**Figure 8.1**). The lesion is isodense, with borders that are difficult to delineate, but it becomes rim-enhancing with administration of contrast. There is a lateral solid component and a medial cystic component. An urgent MRI brain is required.

The MRI scan confirms a large (5 cm by 5 cm) mass in the right hemisphere. It has a heterogeneous solid component and a cystic component medially (**Figure 8.2**). The solid component is relatively hypointense on T1-weighted MRI and hyperintense on T2-weighted MRI and T2–FLAIR. The cystic component is hypointense on T1-weighted MRI and hyperintense on T2-weighted MRI, but is not attenuated on T2–FLAIR, which suggests that the cyst is not in communication with cerebrospinal fluid in the ventricular system.

Diagnosis

The differential diagnosis includes other causes of a rim-enhancing lesion (metastasis, abscess, glioma, infarct, contusion, AIDS-related lesions, lymphoma/lymphoproliferative disorders, demyelination, resolving haeomatoma) The imaging findings, in conjunction with the history, suggest an intrinsic brain tumour, most likely a glioma.

Management

The patient is referred urgently to the neurosurgical registrar. An urgent referral to the neuro-oncology multidisciplinary team is also made. In the meantime, the registrar advises a course of dexamethasone to treat the oedema and reduce the intracranial pressure. A CT chest, abdomen and pelvis is also requested to help exclude an extracranial primary cancer.

The patient undergoes resection of the tumours. Pathological investigation later confirms a glioblastoma.

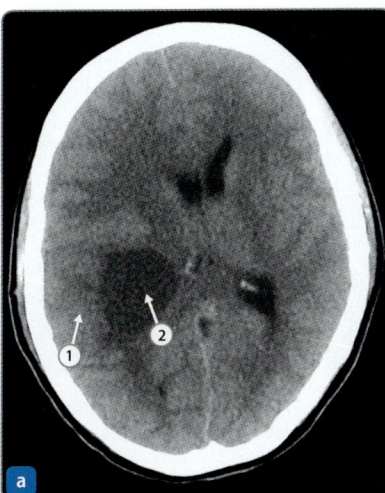

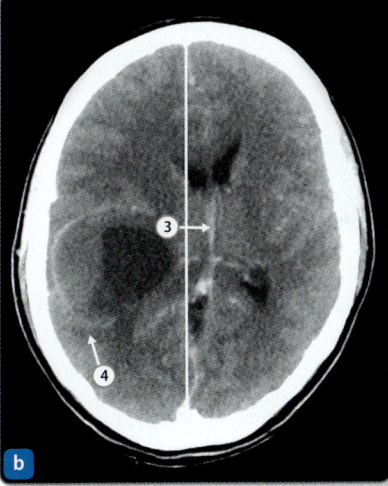

Figure 8.1 Axial CT scan of the head, showing a cerebral mass: (a) before and (b) after administration of contrast. (1) Solid component of the lesion, (2) cystic component of the lesion, (3) midline shift, (4) post-contrast rim enhancement.

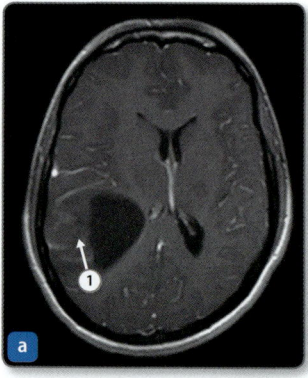

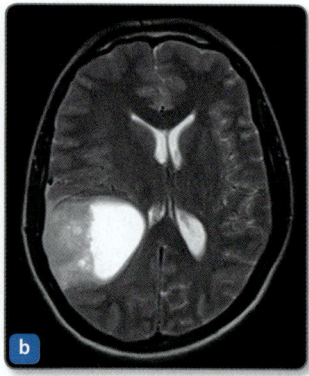

Figure 8.2 Axial MRI scans showing a cerebral mass (same patient as in Figure 8.1): (a) T1-weighted with contrast, (b) T2-weighted and (c) T2–FLAIR. ① Solid component (showing heterogeneity), ② cystic component (with partial attenuation on T2–FLAIR).

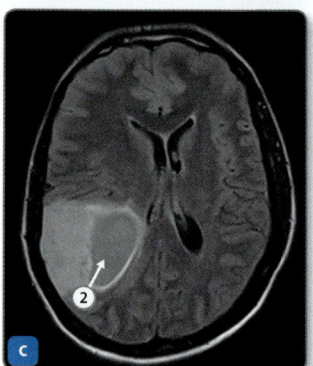

8.2 Approach to the patient with a brain tumour

Assessment

The initial presentation of brain tumours varies, but in most patients, it is a combination of the following:

- Symptoms of increased intracranial pressure:
  - Progressively worsening headache (typically worsened by lying down or coughing)
  - Nausea and vomiting
  - Visual disturbance (caused by papilloedema)

- Focal neurological deficits
- Higher cognitive dysfunction
- Seizures

Some patients present acutely because of the development of intraparenchymal haemorrhage or obstructive hydrocephalus as a result of tumour growth.

Role of neuroimaging

Neuroimaging has become a crucial component in the diagnostic work-up and management of brain tumours.

Note that the diagnosis of a brain tumour is only confirmed on pathological results. Any label given to a lesion before pathological results are obtained is a 'radiological diagnosis' and considered a prediction of the pathology.

CT For patients who present acutely or for whom other causes (e.g. haemorrhage) need to be excluded, a CT of the head is acquired. CT of the chest, abdomen and pelvis is also used, to rule out a primary lesion elsewhere.

MRI This is invariably required in the investigation of suspected brain tumours; compared with other imaging modalities, it offers superior spatial resolution and therefore more detailed visualisation of structures. MRI with contrast is essential, because contrast enhancement enables further prediction of tumour type and grade. In addition, advanced MRI sequences can aid investigation of suspected brain tumours. For example, diffusion-weighted imaging is used to help differentiate brain tumour from cerebral abscess (see section 7.2).

Differential diagnoses

When the results of neuro-imaging show a lesion that might be a tumour, a broad differential diagnosis must be considered. A systematic

> ### Clinical insight
>
> A cerebral abscess should be included as a differential diagnosis if restricted diffusion is apparent on diffusion weighted imaging.

approach to interpretation is used, taking into account the location, number and appearance of any lesions, alongside the clinical context.

Management

Initial management of brain tumours includes the use of steroids, if there is significant oedema causing mass effect, or antiepileptic drugs, if the patient is having seizures. If the patient is acutely unwell, referral to the on-call neurosurgeon is warranted; otherwise, patients are referred urgently to the neuro-oncology service.

The continuing management of brain tumours requires a multidisciplinary approach, with input from neurosurgeons, neurologists, neuro-oncologists, radiologists and specialist nurses. A combination of surgery (to obtain a specimen from biopsy or resection), radiotherapy and chemotherapy are used. Each patient requires an individualised approach, depending on the following factors:

- The diagnosis (i.e. the type of brain tumour)
- The location of the tumour (and its proximity to functionally important structures)
- The general health of the patient (their premorbid state and functional status).

8.3 Glioma

Gliomas are tumours derived from the glial cells in the normal brain, i.e. astrocytes, oligodendrocytes, ependymal cells and microglia. They are graded I–IV, according to the World Health Organization (WHO) system (**Table 8.1**). Grades I and II are referred to as low-grade glioma, and grades III and IV as high-grade glioma. Grade is determined by histopathological findings. However, features found on imaging may also help predict whether a glioma is low or high grade.

Gliomas arise from the tissue of the brain itself and are therefore referred to as intrinsic or intra axial brain tumours.

Low-grade glioma

Low-grade gliomas are those classified as WHO grade I or II.

Key facts

- Compared with high-grade gliomas, low-grade gliomas tend to occur in younger patients, and these patients have a better prognosis

Low- or high-grade category	WHO grade	Example(s)
Low grade	I	Pilocytic astrocytoma Subependymoma
	II	Diffuse astrocytoma Oligodendroglioma Ependymoma
High grade	III	Anaplastic astrocytoma Anaplastic oligodendroglioma Anaplastic ependymoma
	IV	Glioblastoma (astrocytoma)

Table 8.1 World Health Organization (WHO) classification of glioma

- Seizures as a first presentation is more common in low-grade glioma than in high-grade glioma
- Low grade gliomas transform into high grade gliomas in a minority of cases

Imaging findings
- On pathological examination, low grade gliomas extend further than the margin between brain and tumour shown on imaging
- Evidence of calcification is more often present in cases of oligodendroglioma
- Contrast enhancement on either CT or MRI is uncommon but often occurs in oligodendrogliomas

CT In most cases, a low-grade glioma appears as a hypo- or isodense, homogeneous structure on CT, with no contrast enhancement.

MRI On MRI, a low-grade glioma appears as a homogenous structure with no contrast enhancement (**Figure 8.3**). It tends to be hypointense on T1-weighted MRI and hyperintense on T2-weighted MRI.

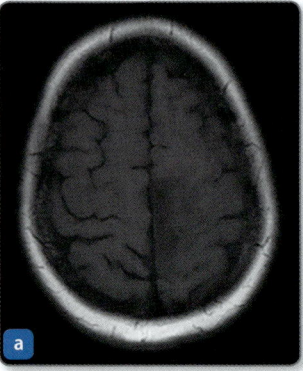
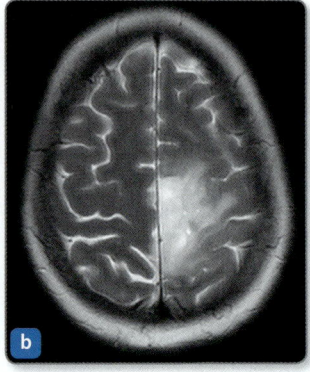

Figure 8.3 MRI scan showing a left frontoparietal low-grade glioma: (a) T1-weighted, (b) T2-weighted and (c) T2–FLAIR.

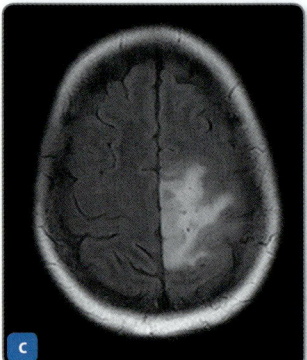

High-grade glioma

High-grade gliomas are WHO grade III or IV.

Key facts

- Glioblastoma (previously termed glioblastoma multiforme) is a grade IV glioma, which is an astrocytoma. Glioblastoma is the most common primary intrinsic brain tumour in adults, and has a poor prognosis
- High-grade gliomas arise either de novo or secondary to transformation of low-grade gliomas

Imaging findings

- High-grade gliomas have distinctive features when compared with low-grade gliomas:
    - High-grade gliomas are more likely to be contrast-enhancing
    - High-grade gliomas are more heterogeneous, meaning that different areas of the tumour appear different (e.g. some areas may enhance contrast, whereas others do not)
- The invasive nature of these tumours causes disruption of the blood–brain barrier, resulting in vasogenic oedema and mass effect
- Glioblastoma may show even further heterogeneity, central necrosis and cystic components (**Figure 8.4**)

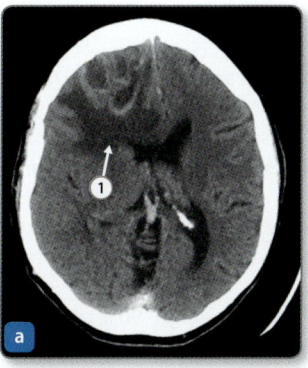
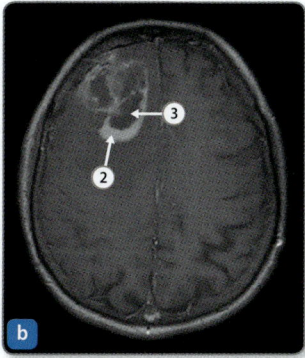
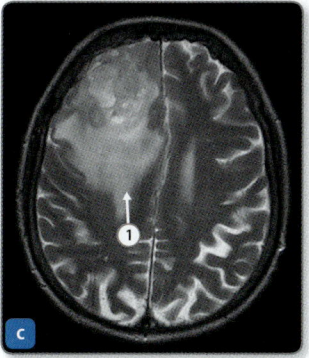

Figure 8.4 Axial CT and MRI scans showing a right frontal glioblastoma: (a) CT (post contrast), (b) T1-weighted MRI (post contrast) and (c) T2-weighted MRI. ① Vasogenic oedema, ② contrast-enhancing component, ③ central necrosis.

CT High-grade glioma often appears as a hypo- or isodense, heterogeneous lesion that is rim-enhancing with contrast. Vasogenic oedema often surrounds the tumour and appears as hypodensity on CT.

MRI High-grade glioma appears hypointense on T1-weighted MRI and hyperintense on T2-weighted MRI. Rim enhancement is seen on T1-weighted MRI with contrast. Vasogenic oedema appears hypointense on T1-weighted MRI and hyperintense on T2-weighted MRI.

8.4 Meningioma

A meningioma is a tumour derived from the dura mater of the meninges.

Key facts
- In contrast to glioma, meningiomas are extra-axial (external to the brain parenchyma), and mostly benign
- The main risk factors are increasing age, female sex, obesity, radiation exposure and certain rare syndromes (e.g. neurofibromatosis)
- Most meningiomas are dural-based (attached to the dura mater) and can therefore occur at any site where there is dura, including the skull base
- Meningiomas are graded as WHO I (benign; 90% of cases), II (atypical; 10%) and III (malignant; < 1%)
- Most patients will present with a combination of symptoms (e.g. raised intracranial pressure, seizures, focal neurological deficit, higher cognitive dysfunction) or the meningioma may be an incidental finding in an asymptomatic patient

Imaging findings
- Meningiomas are extra-axial, and in many cases this is made evident by identification of a 'cerebrospinal fluid cleft' (a rim of fluid between the tumour and the brain parenchyma)
- Meningiomas are generally well-defined and homogeneous lesions
- Meningiomas are in confluence with the meninges

- They enhance strongly and uniformly after administration of contrast
- They may show calcification, suggesting that the tumour has been growing slowly for many years
- Extradural extension and erosion of the skull may also occur in some cases

CT Meningiomas appear iso- or hyperdense (**Figure 8.5a**). They enhance vividly with contrast.

MRI Meningiomas appear hypo- to isointense on T1-weighted MRI and iso- to hyperintense on T2-weighted MRI (**Figures 8.5b** and **c**, and **8.6**). They enhance vividly on T1-weighted MRI.

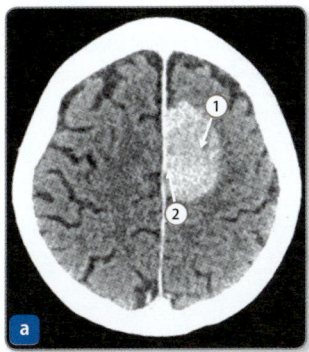
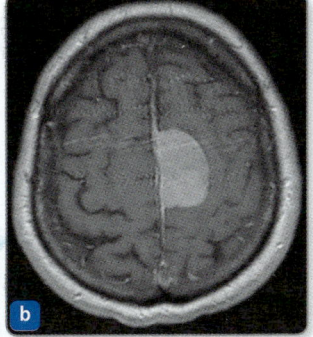
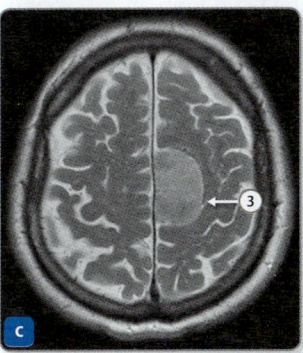

Figure 8.5 CT and MRI scans showing a left parasagittal meningioma: (a) CT (post contrast), (b) T1-weighted MRI (post contrast) and (c) T2-weighted MRI. (1) Vividly enhancing meningioma, (2) dural attachment, (3) cerebrospinal fluid cleft sign.

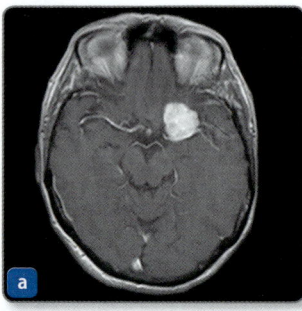

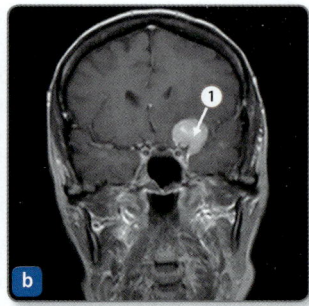

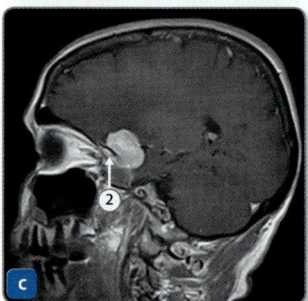

Figure 8.6 T1-weighted MRI scan (post contrast) showing a meningioma of the clinoid process: (a) axial, (b) coronal and (c) sagittal. ① Homogeneous enhancement of the meningioma, ② dural attachment to the skull base.

8.5 Brain metastases

Brain metastases are secondary brain tumours, i.e. those that have spread (metastasised) to the brain from an extracranial primary site. They are the most common form of brain tumour.

Key facts

- Metastases most commonly spread from the lung, breast, skin (melanoma), kidneys or bowel
- Clinical presentation varies, and follows much the same pattern as glioma and meningioma
- If the primary cancer is unknown, and especially in cases in which one or more secondary brain tumours are suspected, a CT of the chest, abdomen and pelvis is considered to search for the primary tumour

Imaging findings

- Brain metastases can be solitary lesions (**Figure 8.7**), but in most cases, multiple lesions are present
- In adults, primary brain tumours tend to be supratentorial (superior to the tentorium cerebelli), but brain metastases are often infratentorial (inferior to the tentorium cerebelli)
- On both CT and MRI, brain metastases tend to appear as contrast-enhancing lesions, frequently associated with a disproportionate amount of oedema for their size
- Metastases tend to be located at the border between grey and white matter

CT Brain metastases vary in density. However, they tend to be well defined and surrounded by extensive hypodensity (representing vasogenic oedema).

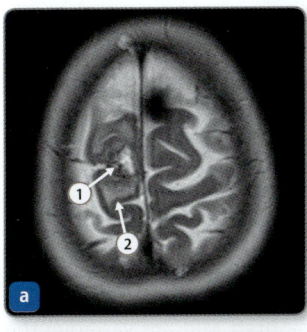

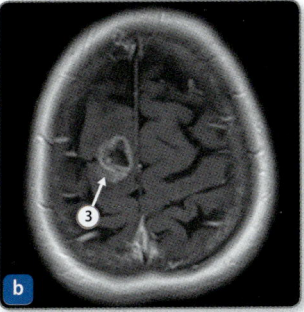

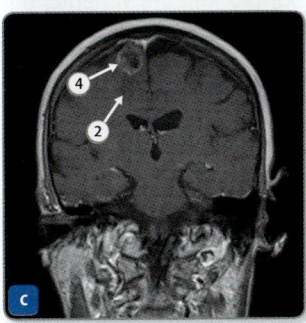

Figure 8.7 MRI scans showing a solitary metastasis in the right posterior frontal lobe in a patient with previously known breast cancer: (a) Axial T2-weighted, (b) axial T1-weighted (post contrast) and (c) coronal T1-weighted (post contrast). ① Solitary metastasis showing heterogeneity, ② vasogenic oedema, ③ rim enhancement with contrast, ④ metastasis at the grey–white matter boundary.

MRI Brain metastases typically appear hypointense on T1-weighted MRI and hyperintense on T2-weighted MRI. They are rim-enhancing with contrast (**Figure 8.7**).

8.6 Pituitary adenoma

A sellar tumour is one occupying the sellar turcica, the depression in the skull base within which lies the hypophyseal fossa, which holds the pituitary gland.

Pituitary adenoma is the most commonly occurring sellar mass.

Key facts

• Pituitary tumours are classified according to size, i.e. microadenomas (< 10 mm) versus macroadenomas (> 10 mm)
• They are also classified by hormonal status, i.e. hormonally active (secretory) versus inactive (non-secretory)
• Pituitary adenomas present with symptoms of hormonal imbalance (either over- or underactivity), the symptoms of compression of adjacent structures (e.g. damage to the optic chiasm, causing bitemporal hemianopia) or pituitary apoplexy haemorrhage into or infarction of the pituitary gland

Imaging findings

Pituitary adenomas are best visualised on MRI.

MRI Pituitary adenomas appear isointense to grey matter on T1-weighted MRI, and are typically contrast enhancing (**Figure 8.8**). Findings on T2-weighted MRI are variable; the adenoma appears either isointense or hyperintense to the grey matter.

Microadenomas can be subtle. Thin-slice MRI is needed when an adenoma is suspected. Macroadenomas are seen to emerge from the sellar turcica but are restricted and narrowed at its roof (the diaphragm). Areas of necrosis, haemorrhage or cysts are often visible in large, macroadenomas.

Management

Management of pituitary tumours requires the input of a neurosurgeon, an endocrinologist and an ophthalmologist. Tumour size, hormone status and symptoms determine whether observation or treatment with either medical hormone therapy or surgery (e.g. trans-sphenoidal hypophysectomy) is most appropriate.

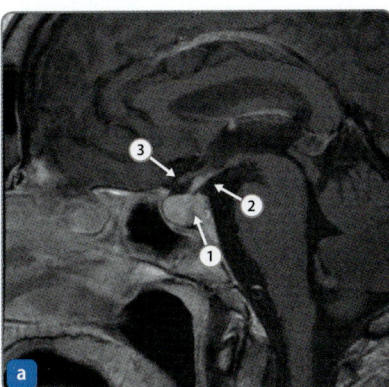

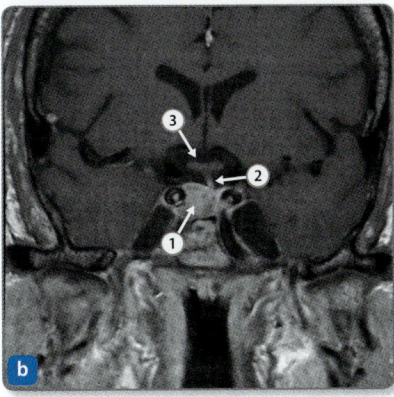

Figure 8.8 T1-weighted MRI scan with contrast, showing pituitary macroadenoma: (a) sagittal and (b) coronal. (1) Pituitary gland and macroadenoma (12 mm by 12 mm), (2) infundibulum (pituitary stalk), (3) optic chiasm.

8.7 Medulloblastoma

Medulloblastoma is a common brain tumour in children.

Key facts

- Unlike ependymoma and astrocytoma, which are derived from neuroepithelial cells, medulloblastoma is derived from embryonal cells
- Medulloblastoma arises in the cerebellum, therefore patients present with cerebellar dysfunction or symptoms and signs of increased intracranial pressure (owing to obstructive hydrocephalus)
- Medulloblastomas may communicate with the ventricles or subarachnoid space, therefore a full spine MRI scan is required to exclude distant progression

Imaging findings

MRI Medulloblastoma appears as a midline or paramedian mass. These tumours are hypointense on T1-weighted MRI, and hyperintense, yet heterogeneous, on T2-weighted MRI. Sites of necrosis, cystic components and haemorrhage are often present. Most medulloblastomas are contrast-enhancing.

Obstructive hydrocephalus may be present if the fourth ventricle is effaced.

8.8 Vestibular schwannoma

A vestibular schwannoma (also known as an acoustic neuroma) is a benign tumour that arises from the eighth cranial nerve (the vestibulocochlear nerve).

Key facts

- Vestibular schwannoma typically presents with hearing loss, tinnitus, imbalance or facial weakness
- Obstructive hydrocephalus occurs when large vestibular schwannomas efface the fourth ventricle.
- A rare syndrome called neurofibromatosis type 2 is associated with bilateral vestibular schwannoma
- Differential diagnoses include ependymoma, meningioma and metastasis

Imaging findings

MRI Vestibular schwannomas are in the cerebellopontine angle and typically include an intracanalicular component. They usually appear as a solid nodular mass but often include a cystic component (**Figure 8.9**).

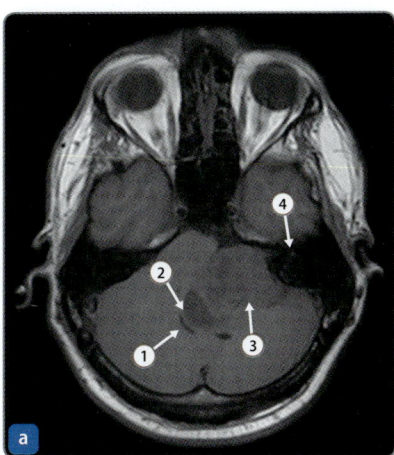

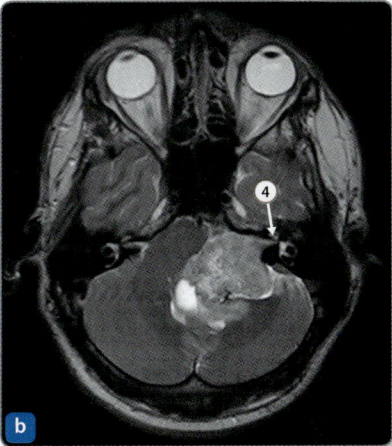

Figure 8.9 Axial MRI scans showing a left vestibular schwannoma: (a) T1-weighted, (b) T2-weighted. ① Effacement of the fourth ventricle, ② cystic component, ③ solid component, ④ intracanalicular spread.

Compared with surrounding parenchyma, the solid component of a vestibular schwannoma appears hypo- or isointense on T1-weighted MRI, and hyperintense on T2-weighted MRI. The cystic component is hypointense on T1-weighted MRI (but occasionally poorly differentiated from the solid component), and hyperintense on T2-weighted MRI. Most vestibular schwannomas are contrast-enhancing.

8.9 Image-guided neurosurgery

In recent decades, the surgical treatment of brain tumours has undergone the technological advances of image-guided neurosurgery ('neuronavigation'). The principles of these new techniques also apply to neurosurgery for other conditions.

Stereotactic surgery

Stereotactic surgery is an image-guided, minimally invasive technique. A frame is mounted to the head of the patient, and then both the patient and the frame are scanned. With the head and frame within the same imaging volume, the target lesion can be localised in relation to the frame. Using the coordinates for the target lesion, a safe trajectory is planned.

This technique is used to obtain biopsy specimens from lesions such as brain tumours. Other applications are ablation of lesions and neurostimulation (e.g. deep brain stimulation for movement disorders, such as Parkinson's disease).

Frameless image guidance

Advancements in stereotactic neurosurgery have led to development of a frameless technique for obtaining biopsy specimens. Either CT or MRI is used to map landmarks of the head in a three-dimensional space. Using a sensor next to the patient and a probe with a sensor (often termed a wand), these landmarks can be identified in real time without the need for frame.

Advanced image guidance

Resection of lesions (e.g. tumours or epileptic foci) poses risks to important brain regions. Several advanced techniques have been developed to locate functionally important anatomical areas of the brain, and thereby facilitate attempts to avoid damage to these regions and preserve function.

Functional MRI This is used to investigate the proximity of brain tumours to important brain structures. The results are used to inform the decision on whether surgery is possible, and if surgery is carried out, to avoid causing iatrogenic neurological deficits.

Tractography In the diffusion MRI technique known as tractography (or fibre tracking), the directionality of water movement is used to predict the arrangement of white matter tracts (**Figure 8.10**). Tractography is used to plan surgical approaches that spare these tracts; for example, vision is preserved by sparing the optic radiation.

Intraoperative imaging

Only a few neurosurgical units in the UK have an intraoperative MRI scanner. Intraoperative MRI allows surgeons to update

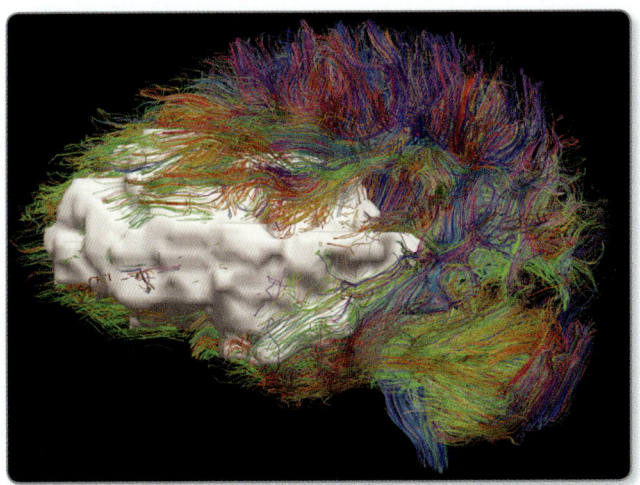

Figure 8.10 Tractography (fibre tracking). Courtesy of Dr M Bastin, Edinburgh, UK.

neuronavigation data as a procedure progresses. They then use the information to correct their surgical approach for brain shift (when the anatomy of the brain changes once resection begins), and to review the extent of tumour resection before continuing.

An intraoperative MRI theatre either has an MRI scanner that slides along tracks towards the operating table, or an operating table that moves towards an MRI scanner.

Spinal conditions

Spinal conditions are pathologies affecting the vertebrae and spinal cord. There are several broad groups:

- Trauma
- Degeneration
- Inflammation (see Chapter 6)
- Infection (see Chapter 7)
- Tumours
- Congenital abnormality
- Vascular disease

9.1 Clinical scenario

Cauda equina syndrome

Presentation

A 45-year-old woman attends her general practice urgently after experiencing a 48-hour history of progressively worsening back pain, bilateral leg weakness and loss of sensation in her legs. She has had minor back pain for the previous 10 years, but it has never been so severe. On further questioning, she admits that she was incontinent of urine that morning. On examination, the patient has bilateral weakness of ankle dorsiflexion, a bilateral sensory level of L5, saddle paraesthesia and loss of anal tone.

The general practitioner makes an urgent referral to the nearest neurosurgical department and arranges for the patient to be admitted.

Initial interpretation

The combination of leg weakness, the pattern of paraesthesia, and urinary incontinence makes the clinical diagnosis of cauda equina syndrome. This is a neurosurgical emergency. Urgent MRI of the spine is required to investigate the cause. Only an MRI scan can confirm or exclude the diagnosis definitively.

Imaging findings

The MRI lumbar spine shows multilevel intervertebral disc herniation, but only one disc herniation (at L4–L5) is compressing the cauda equina (**Figure 9.1**).

Diagnosis

The finding of a herniated L4–L5 intervertebral disc corresponds with the clinical diagnosis of cauda equina syndrome.

Management

Once a diagnosis of cauda equina syndrome has been made, the patient should immediately undergo urgent surgical

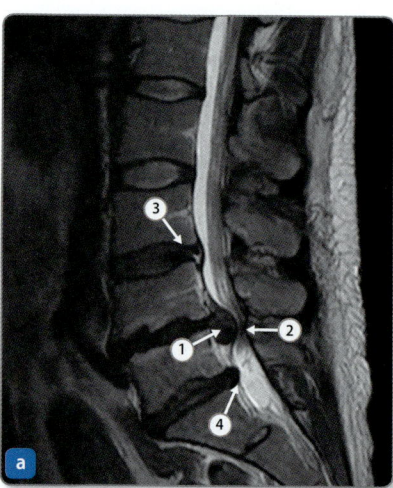

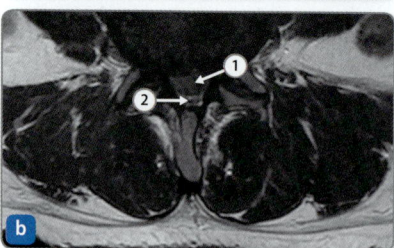

Figure 9.1 T2-weighted MRI scans from a patient with cauda equina syndrome: (a) sagittal, (b) axial (at the L4–L5 level). ① L4–L5 intervertebral disc herniation, ② compression of the cauda equina at the L4–L5 level. There are two small, non-compressive disc herniations at L3–L4 ③ and L5–S1 ④.

decompression and discectomy to try to prevent the development of permanent neurological deficit.

9.2 Approach to the patient with spinal trauma

With spinal trauma, the spinal cord must be protected from further injury. Therefore, a precautionary approach is always used. Until the potential for further injury can be assessed, three-point immobilisation (collar, blocks and tape) is used to prevent movement of the cervical spine. All other spinal precautions are required; for example, the log-rolling technique is used to turn the patient while keeping their spine in alignment.

Computerised tomography of the cervical spine is the definitive investigation for suspected or possible cervical column injury. In patients who have sustained a head injury, indications for CT imaging within 1 hour, according to current UK guidelines, are:
- Clinical suspicion of an injury in the alert and stable patient, and any one of the following:
  - A dangerous mechanism
  - Presence of a neurological deficit
  - Patient's age 65 years or older
- A Glasgow Coma Scale score less than 13 (see chapter 4) or use of intubation
- Suspicious or abnormal cervical spine radiograph
- An adequate cervical spine radiograph is not attainable
- A multiregion CT 'trauma series' scan is being obtained

Plain radiographs of the cervical spine are obtained for conscious patients for whom there are no indications for CT imaging, but who have neck pain or tenderness and restriction of neck rotation. If an injury is detected on plain radiography, CT imaging is needed for further assessment.

Clinical insight

Cervical spine injury is a concern in unconscious patients presenting with head injury. If it is not recognised, treatment is delayed and there is a risk of the development or worsening of neurological deficits.

Patients with neurological deficits require further assessment with MRI. Suspected discoligamentous injuries also require MRI.

All imaging is carried out with the cervical spine protection kept on and with the spinal precautions adhered to.

9.3 Spinal fractures

Spinal fractures are mostly due to trauma, but pathological fractures (e.g. a fracture caused by malignancy) also occur. Fractures affect any of the cervical, thoracic, lumbar, sacral or coccygeal vertebrae. Fractures range from those that have no consequence and do not need intervention, to those that damage the spinal cord and need surgical intervention.

Cervical spine fractures

Because of its mobility and comparative lack of soft tissue protection, the cervical spine is the most commonly injured part of the spine in trauma.

Key facts

- A **Jefferson's fracture** is a burst fracture of the atlas (C1). It is typically caused by axial loading, for example as a result of the patient falling and landing head first. Fracture lines are visible in both the anterior and posterior elements, and occasionally extend into the lateral masses. The lateral masses become displaced; this is best appreciated on an odontoid view radiograph or on CT
- A **hangman's fracture** is a bilateral pars (pars interarticularis) fracture of C2, which if there is associated rupture of the C2–C3 disc, can result in subluxation of C2 on C3 (**Figure 9.2**)
- An **odontoid fracture** (fracture of the odontoid process) is typically caused by hyperflexion. It is usually stable, particularly if it has occurred in the context of a low-velocity injury in an elderly patient. It can be diagnosed using the odontoid view on plain radiography (**Figure 9.3**). Odontoid fractures can be classified using the Anderson and D'Alonzo system into those that involve the odontoid process (tip or base) and those that extend to the lateral masses

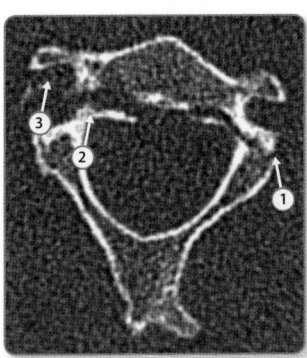

Figure 9.2 Axial CT scan (bone window) showing a hangman's fracture (of C2). There is fracture of both the left ① and right ② pars, with involvement of the transverse foramen on the right ③.

- A **flexion teardrop fracture** is caused by hyperflexion and can be unstable. There is avulsion of the anterior corner of the vertebral body. This is caused by avulsion, by the anterior longitudinal ligament, of a fragment of bone from the vertebral body. In associated posterior column injury, anterior subluxation of a vertebral body (anterolisthesis) can occur and the spinal cord is at risk of being injured (**Figure 9.4**)
- A **facet fracture** is caused by hyperextension and can be unstable. Facet fractures can be unilateral or bilateral. A bifacet dislocation is highly unstable and often leads to ventral subluxation with spinal cord injury, requiring urgent reduction and fixation (**Figure 9.5**)

Imaging findings

Plain radiography

Three views of the cervical spine are routinely obtained: antero-posterior, lateral and odontoid. The cervical spine radiographs are systematically screened for injury, as described in Chapter 2. Chapter 2 describes the normal spine, and should be read before trying to interpret the images of the abnormal spine presented in this chapter.

On a plain radiograph, a fracture or injury is suspected in the presence of:

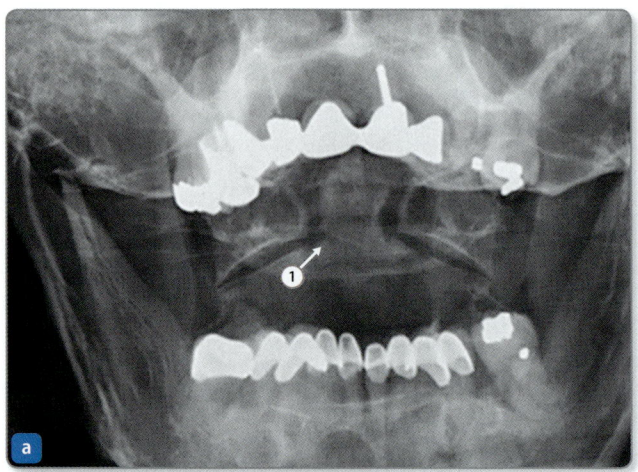

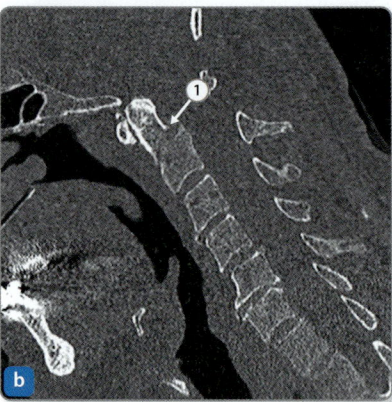

Figure 9.3 Odontoid plain radiograph (a) and sagittal CT (bone window) (b) showing an odontoid fracture. ① The fracture line.

- An obvious fracture line or detachment of bone (e.g. a spinous process fracture)
- Loss of structural integrity (change in shape and size) of the vertebral components
- Loss of normal alignment
- Loss of normal and equal distance between structures

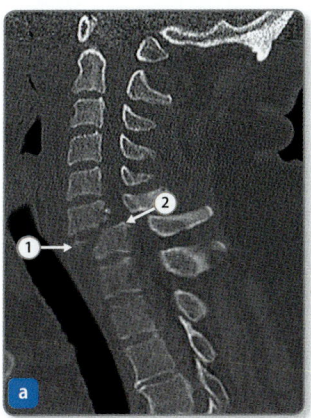 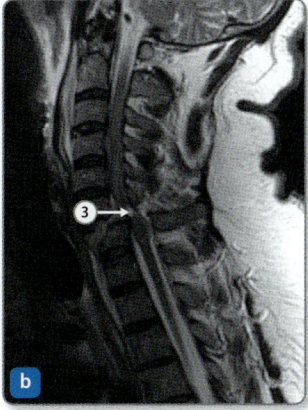

Figure 9.4 (a) Sagittal CT scan (bone window) and (b) sagittal T2-weighted MRI scan showing a flexion teardrop fracture. ① Avulsion of the anterior corner of the C7 vertebral body, ② dislocation of C6 on C7, ③ transection of the spinal cord.

Note that cervical spine radiographs can appear completely normal even with significant injury. If there is a high suspicion or high risk of injury, CT is required.

CT This is the principal imaging modality for investigating cervical spine injuries, because it offers cross-sectional views of the spinal column in the axial, sagittal and coronal planes. These are essential for radiological assessment of an injury.

MRI This is required when there is a suspicion of a discoligamentous injury, or to investigate the integrity of the spinal cord if the patient has a neurological deficit.

Management

Patients with a confirmed cervical spine fracture require full spinal precautions initially, including cervical spine protection (three-point immobilisation). Spinal injuries or fractures in the rest of the spine should be considered. Management of cervical spine fracture is discussed with a neurosurgeon or spinal orthopaedic surgeon.

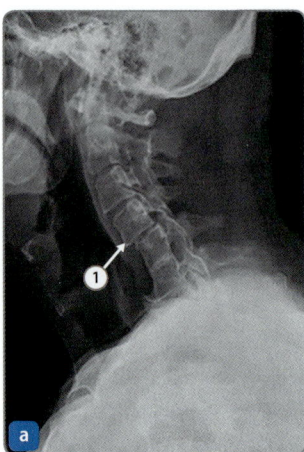

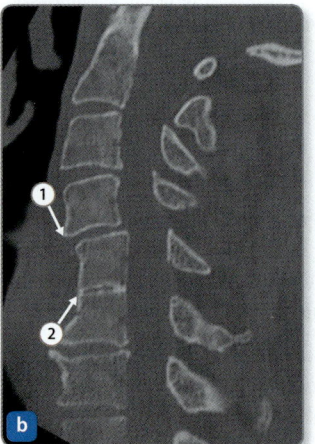

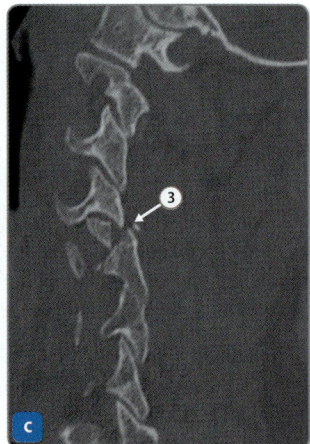

Figure 9.5 (a) Lateral plain radiograph and (b and c) sagittal CT scans (bone window) showing a displaced fracture of the left facet joint of C4, causing anterolisthesis of the C4 body on C5. There is incidental fusion of the C5 and C6 bodies. ① Displacement of C4 on C5 (anterolisthesis), ② fusion of the C5–C6 vertebral bodies, ③ fracture of the left facet joint of C4.

Thoracolumbar fractures

Most thoracolumbar fractures occur at the thoracolumbar junction (T12–L1), because this part of the spine lies between the relatively immobile thoracic spine and the more mobile lumbar spine.

Key facts

- A **wedge (or compression) fracture** is common in elderly patients, who are preferentially affected by osteoporosis. It is often termed a fragility fracture, because it is caused by low-energy trauma. However, it can also occur in hyperflexion injuries. Wedge fractures are most common in the lumbar spine. There is wedge-like compression of the anterior vertebral body, loss of vertebral height and increased kyphosis of the spine (**Figure 9.7**). Anterior wedge fractures are considered stable, because they typically include only the anterior column

- A **burst fracture** is typically the result of vertical compression, and both the anterior and middle columns are involved. Burst fractures are often unstable. Part of the vertebral body

> ### Clinical insight
>
> An injury of the vertebrae can be described as stable or unstable. Denis' three-column theory is one method that surgeons use to assess the potential for further displacement (**Figure 9.6**).

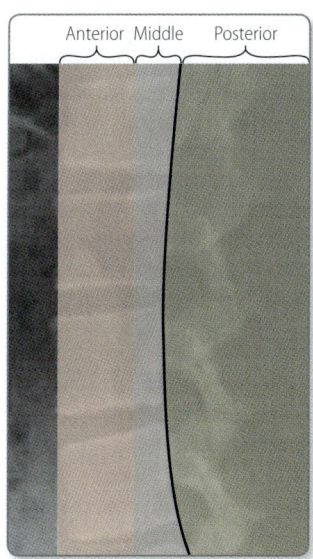

Anterior Middle   Posterior

Figure 9.6 Denis' three-column theory of stability. Generally, if two or more columns are injured, the fracture is considered unstable. The anterior column consists of the anterior two thirds of the vertebral body and the anterior longitudinal ligament. The middle column consists of the posterior third of the vertebral body, the posterior longitudinal ligament and the posterior part of the annular fibrosis. The posterior column consists of the remaining posterior vertebral components.

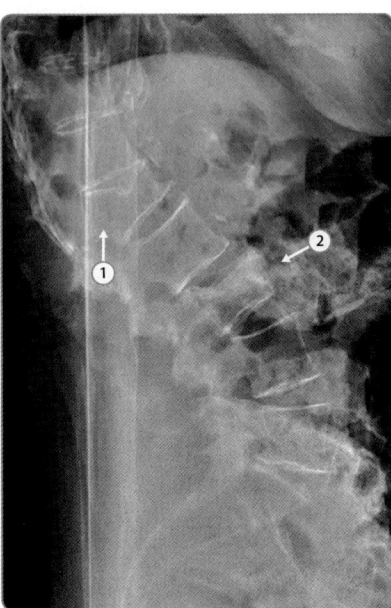

Figure 9.7 Lateral plain radiograph of the lumbar spine, showing wedge compression fractures at L1 (1) and L3 (2).

may be displaced posteriorly into the spinal canal, thereby compressing the spinal cord or cauda equina (**Figure 9.8**)

Imaging findings

The general imaging principles described for cervical spine fractures also hold true for thoracolumbar fractures. A description of how to interpret images of the normal thoracolumbar spine and systematically search for fractures is provided in section 2.3.

Management

Thoracolumbar fractures, particularly in the absence of neurological involvement, are mostly managed initially with bed rest. If one part of the spine is known to have a fracture, images of the rest of the spine are obtained to exclude others.

An expert spinal opinion is sought regarding the management of these injuries. Patients with neurological deficits require urgent MRI and may require surgical intervention.

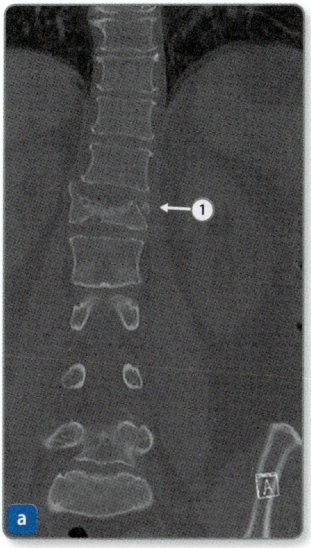
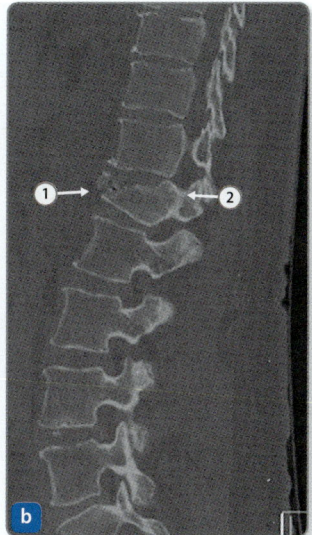
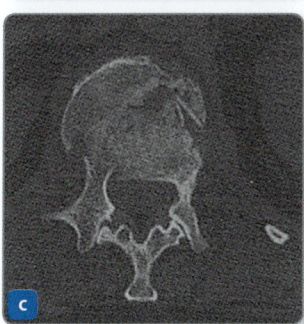

Figure 9.8 CT scan (bone window) showing an L1 burst fracture: (a) coronal, (b) sagittal and (c) axial. The fracture involves the anterior and middle columns of L1 ①, causing loss of height and retropulsion of the superior–posterior corner of the vertebral body ②.

9.4 Degenerative spinal conditions

As the average age of the UK population continues to rise, degenerative conditions, including those affecting the spine, have become increasingly common. Degeneration of the intervertebral discs and associated soft tissues cause structural changes that impinge on and can result in compression of the spinal cord and nerve roots.

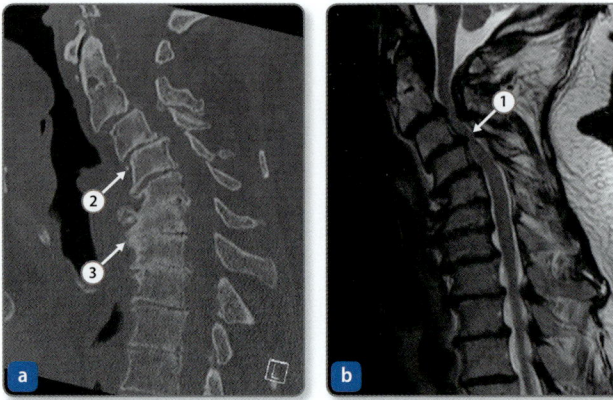

Figure 9.9 (a) Sagittal CT scan (bone window) and (b) sagittal T2-weighted MRI scan (b) showing cervical stenosis causing cervical myelopathy. ① Stenosis of the spinal canal, ② spondylolisthesis of C2–C4, ③ loss of disc space.

Common features of spinal degeneration are:
- Intervertebral disc herniation (discussed later in this section)
- Osteophytes (abnormal new bone growth)
- Hypertrophy of facet joints
- Hypertrophy of ligaments (especially the ligamentum flavum)

These changes usually result in slowly progressive syndromes, such as spinal stenosis causing myelopathy (**Figure 9.9**).

Intervertebral disc herniation

Herniation occurs when a structure is abnormally displaced into another anatomical space. Disc herniation (or prolapse) occurs when the inner nucleus pulposus of the intervertebral disc herniates through the outer annulus fibrosis.

Key facts

- Intervertebral discs tend to herniate posterolaterally, thereby compressing the nerve root, with consequent clinical symptoms and signs of radiculopathy

- Central disc herniation causes compression of the spinal cord above the conus medullaris (typically at L1) or of the cauda equina below the conus medullaris (see **Figure 9.1**)
- Herniation can occur at any level but is most common in the lumbar spine

Imaging findings

MRI The intervertebral discs are best visualised on MRI in both sagittal and axial views. A normal intervertebral disc has intermediate to high signal on T2-weighted MRI, but ageing discs become hypointense on T2-weighted MRI.

Disc herniation can cause foraminal lateral recess or central canal narrowing with associated neural compression, if the prolapse is large enough.

> ### Clinical insight
>
> **Spondylosis** is a non-specific term for degenerative changes of the spine. Spondylotic features include intervertebral disc herniation, osteophytes, hypertrophic facets and ligamentous hypertrophy.
>
> **Spondylolysis** describes a defect in the pars interarticularis of the vertebra.
>
> **Spondylolisthesis** describes the translation of one vertebral body on the one below. This can be congenital, degenerative or acquired secondary to trauma (as discussed earlier in this chapter).

Management

If disc herniation causes acute spinal cord compression or cauda equina syndrome, urgent surgical decompression is required.

The natural history of disc herniation causing either cervical or lumbar radiculopathy is favourable, and most patients can be treated conservatively with analgesia and rest. By 3 months, 70% of patients, and by 1 year, 95%, are pain-free. Surgery is reserved for patients with prolonged disabling symptoms or in severe pain. There is no evidence that early surgery for foot drop results in a better outcome, compared with the natural history.

9.5 Spinal tumours

Spinal tumours are classified as extradural or intradural. Intradural tumours are further divided into extramedullary tumours, which form outside the spinal cord parenchyma, and intramedullary tumours, which form within the spinal cord parenchyma (**Table 9.1**).

Primary spinal tumours are derived from cells of the spinal cord and associated structures. Metastatic (secondary) spinal tumours have spread to the vertebrae from a primary site elsewhere in the body.

Spinal meningioma

A spinal meningioma is an example of an intradural, extramedullary tumour. It involves the dura, from which it arises, outside the spinal cord parenchyma.

Key facts

- Spinal meningiomas are far less common than those that arise within the cranium
- Women in their 50s are most commonly affected
- Patients present with development of progressive neurological deficits, most commonly paraparesis, with the sensory level determined by the spinal level affected

Imaging findings

MRI Spinal meningiomas appear on MRI as well-circumscribed lesions that are adjacent to and may compress the spinal cord (**Figure 9.10**). They most commonly arise in the thoracic spine. Their intensity is variable on T1- and T2-weighted MRI, but they are usually avidly contrast-enhancing

Spinal tumour type	Example(s)
Extradural	Metastasis
Intradural	
Extramedullary	Meningioma
	Nerve sheath tumour
Intramedullary	Glioma (most commonly ependymoma)

Table 9.1 Classification of spinal tumours

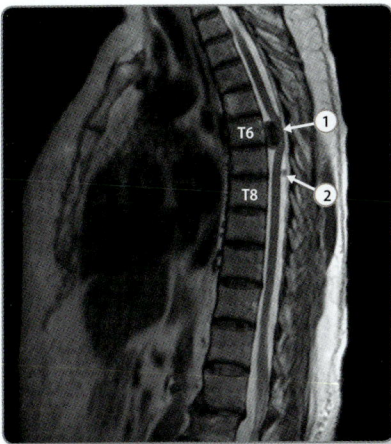

Figure 9.10 Sagittal MRI of the thoracic spine (T2W) demonstrating a meningioma ① at T6 level and a smaller meningioma ② at T7–T8 level.

and are occasionally calcified. There is dural attachment and often a visible dural tail.

Management

Surgical resection is required to prevent further neurological deficit. Recurrence is uncommon if complete resection is achieved. If there is incomplete resection, postoperative radiotherapy is considered.

Spinal ependymoma

A spinal ependymoma is an example of an intradural, intramedullary tumour, because it arises within the spinal cord.

Key facts

- Spinal gliomas are far less common than intracranial gliomas
- Ependymomas account for about 70% of spinal gliomas
- Spinal ependymomas tend to present in patients in their thirties and forties
- Patients present with back pain that typically precedes the development of focal neurological deficit according to the level of the tumour

Imaging findings

MRI Any level of the spinal cord may be affected, with the ependymoma visible as a well-circumscribed lesion in the centre of the cord (**Figure 9.11**). Ependymomas appear hypointense on T1-weighted MRI and hyperintense on T2-weighted MRI. They typically enhance with contrast.

A cavity commonly develops at the superior and sometimes inferior pole of the tumour.

Management

Surgical resection is carried out to prevent the development of further neurological deficit. The prognosis is good when complete resection is achieved, with recurrence rare and often delayed for several decades.

Metastatic spinal cord compression

When metastatic tumours compress the spinal cord, the term metastatic spinal cord compression is used. Metastatic

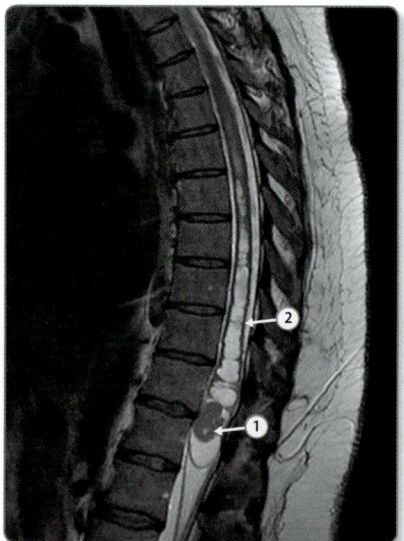

Figure 9.11 Sagittal T2-weighted MRI scan showing an intradural, intramedullary tumour of the spine – an ependymoma ①. The syrinx ② extends superiorly.

compression of the cauda equina results in cauda equina syndrome, as described previously.

Key facts

- The spine is vulnerable to metastases, because it is surrounded by an extensive venous anastomosis that provides a haematogenous route for metastasis
- The thoracic vertebrae are most commonly affected, followed by the lumbar and cervical vertebrae. However, multilevel involvement is common
- The tumours that commonly cause metastatic spinal cord compression include those of the prostate, breast, kidney and lung
- The primary cancer may or may not have already been diagnosed when a patient presents with metastatic spinal cord compression

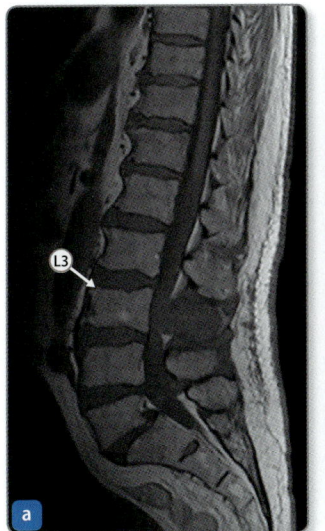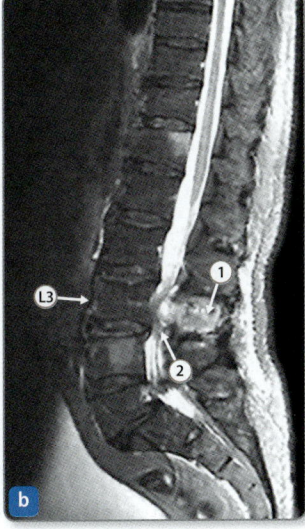

Figure 9.12 MRI scans of the lumbar spine, showing malignant spinal cord compression: (a) sagittal T1-weighted and (b) sagittal T2-weighted. ① Multilevel metastatic lesions involving most severely the posterior elements of the L3 vertebra, ② compression of the cauda equina.

- Pain is a common early symptom, followed by development of neurological deficits according to the level (or levels) affected

Imaging findings

MRT of the spine is the gold standard investigation in patients with suspected metastatic spinal cord compression. It should be carried out within 24 hours of presentation. Plain radiography or CT is insufficient, because the results are often falsely reassuring.

MRI Vertebral metastases are extradural lesions. In metastatic spinal cord compression, the mass is seen to compress the spinal cord (**Figure 9.12**). The intensity of the lesion differs depending on the nature of the primary cancer, and whether or not the tumour is osteolytic (bone-eroding) or osteoblastic (bone-forming).

Management

Metastatic spinal cord compression is an oncological emergency. Patients are given steroids (dexamethasone) to reduce oedema. They require either emergency radiotherapy or surgical decompression.

Index

Note: Page numbers in **bold** or *italic* refer to tables or figures respectively.